# CHANGE CONTROL DIET

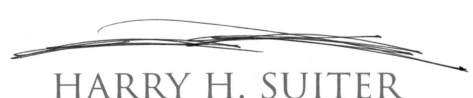

## HARRY H. SUITER

ISBN: 1494228602
ISBN 13: 9781494228606

Library of Congress Control Number: 2013921667
CreateSpace Independent Publishing Platform
North Charleston, South Carolina

# DEDICATION

I dedicate this book to my beautiful wife and two children. My family means everything to me. They give me love, strength, and the motivation to be a better person every day. They have seen me in both good times and bad. Despite the challenge or situation, their love surrounds me always. I would also like to thank two of my mentors, Fred and Martha, for encouraging me to pursue this health program book. I was skeptical that a person without millions of dollars to invest in clinical programs and marketing could make an impact on reducing obesity. Fred and Martha played a critical role in influencing me to self-publish this health program book and believing in me and my potential to help hundreds of millions of people worldwide.

# TABLE OF CONTENTS

# DISCLAIMER

This program should be started with a consultation with a doctor to assess your health and ability to start a new health program. Starting a new health program carries risks that can be minimized under supervision of a doctor. By following this program, you fully accept all responsibility for your own health, your ability to start a new health program, and all risks associated with this program.

# CHAPTER 1

# INTRODUCTION

The weight-loss industry has failed America. The weight-loss industry has failed the world. Though America is the heaviest nation, obesity is a worldwide problem. According to the World Health Organization, here are some astonishing facts on obesity:

- Worldwide obesity has nearly doubled since 1980.

- In 2008, more than 1.4 billion adults, 20 and older, were overweight. Of these over 200 million men and nearly 300 million women were obese.

- 35% of adults aged 20 and over were overweight in 2008, and 11% were obese.

- 65% of the world's population live in countries where overweight and obesity kills more people than underweight.

- More than 40 million children under the age of five were overweight in 2011.

- Obesity is preventable.[1]

Here is an estimate of the number of obese people in the top twenty countries, ranked by millions of obese people per country:[2]

1 http://www.who.int/mediacentre/factsheets/fs311/en/ (World Health Organization, Obesity and Overweight facts)

2 Sources: http://www.worldatlas.com/aatlas/populations/ctypopls.htm (World Atlas, Countries of the World) and http://www.oecd.org/health/49716427.pdf (OECD Organization, Obesity Update 2012)

| Rank | Country | Percent Obese | Population | Number of obese people |
|------|---------|---------------|------------|------------------------|
| 1 | United States | 33.8 | 309,975,000 | 104,771,550 |
| 2 | China | 2.9 | 1,339,190,000 | 38,836,510 |
| 3 | México | 30 | 108,396,211 | 32,518,863 |
| 4 | Brazil | 13.9 | 193,364,000 | 26,877,596 |
| 5 | India | 2.1 | 1,184,639,000 | 24,877,419 |
| 6 | Russia | 16.2 | 141,927,297 | 22,992,222 |
| 7 | United Kingdom | 23 | 62,041,708 | 14,269,593 |
| 8 | Germany | 14.7 | 81,757,600 | 12,018,367 |
| 9 | Turkey | 15.2 | 72,561,312 | 11,029,319 |
| 10 | South Africa | 18.1 | 49,991,300 | 9,048,425 |
| 11 | Canada | 24.2 | 34,207,000 | 8,278,094 |
| 12 | Spain | 16 | 46,951,532 | 7,512,245 |
| 13 | France | 11.2 | 65,447,374 | 7,330,106 |
| 14 | Italy | 10.3 | 60,340,328 | 6,215,054 |
| 15 | Indonesia | 2.4 | 234,181,400 | 5,620,354 |
| 16 | Australia | 24.6 | 22,421,417 | 5,515,669 |
| 17 | Japan | 3.9 | 127,380,000 | 4,967,820 |
| 18 | Poland | 12.5 | 38,167,329 | 4,770,916 |
| 19 | Chile | 25.1 | 17,114,000 | 4,295,614 |
| 20 | Greece | 18.1 | 11,306,183 | 2,046,419 |

Obesity in the period of 1988–1994, as measured by the Centers for Disease Control (CDC), was 22.9 percent for American adults over twenty years of age. From 2009–2010 the obesity percentage rate increased to 35.7 percent of the American population, which is an approximate 50 percent increase. The CDC also measured the number of overweight people (which includes obese people) in the period of 1988–1994 as 56.0 percent. For the period of 2009–2010, this increased to 68.1 percent of the population in the United States. These statistics are eye opening: approximately one out of every three Americans is obese and approximately seven out of ten (including obese people) are overweight. This is equivalent to walking into a room of ten people to find that three people are obese, four people are overweight, and only three people are not overweight.[3]

The weight-loss industry is a multi-billion-dollar industry and is forecasted to reach approximately $41.8 billion in the United States

---

3  http://www.cdc.gov/obesity/data/adult.html (Centers for Disease Control and Prevention, Adult Obesity Facts, 2012)

by 2017, according to RnRMarketResearch.com.[4] The industry is very crowded with exercise programs, food programs, supplements, and gadgets. Weight-loss programs typically advertise very aggressive results in a short period of time—which resulted in the Federal Trade Commission in 2009 requiring companies to remove "Results Not Typical" from advertisements. Hundreds of millions of people are trying to lose weight worldwide. According to a report by ABC, approximately 80 percent of people who lose weight in the United States put the weight back on.[5] I also heard an interesting statistic on the radio one day for the contestants of the hit TV series *The Biggest Loser*: approximately 60 percent of contestants put the weight back on after leaving the show.

I have struggled for more than fifteen years of my life with trying to lose weight. Though I was very skinny as a kid, I put on a lot of weight during my college years and early twenties. This has resulted

4  http://www.prweb.com/releases/weight-management-trends/us-2nd-edition-market/prweb10609499.htm (PRWeb, US Weight Management Market Expected to Reach $41.8 Billion By 2017 in New Research Report at RnRMarketResearch.com, April 2013)
5  http://abcnews.go.com/Health/100-million-dieters-20-billion-weight-loss-industry/story?id=16297197 (ABC News, 100 Million Dieters, $20 Billion: The Weight-Loss Industry by the Numbers, May 2012)

in me bouncing between overweight and obese by medical definition over fifteen years of my life. At five feet eleven inches tall, I was approximately 25–35 pounds overweight and fought the same battle every year. I lost and regained the same 10–15 pounds, which resulted in my weight fluctuating from 210 pounds to 225 pounds throughout the year. I was never able to reach my goal weight of 190 pounds. In addition, my family and friends would get a good laugh out of something I said several times a year: "My diet starts Monday."

I was not alone in this struggle. In fact, *the total sales of the weight-loss industry continue to grow, but there is no reduction in obesity.* One day I decided I would try to understand why. The key thing this fact told me is that the products and programs are failing to connect with the majority of the people who are trying to lose weight. It also suggests that the industry's financial success is thriving on our failures—when we fail, we usually end up buying another program only to fail again. This is great for industry sales; however, it is horrible for the hundreds of millions of people worldwide trying to lose weight.

In my opinion, the industry has failed to reduce obesity because its programs do not focus on how to change human behavior. They assume we are all similar to robots, and we can simply follow the program without emotions, thoughts, and strong cravings for the foods we love. The programs also fail at understanding how to introduce changes to a person's diet and exercise in a controlled manner. Think about it: you can't decide you want to run a marathon tomorrow, so why would think you would be successful changing your habits from eating cheeseburgers and being a "couch potato" to eating salads and exercising in one day? You need to train for a marathon over a long time. It would look something like this: walk a mile, jog a mile, jog two miles, jog three miles, etc., working your way up to 26.2 miles over a long period. Another way to relate to this concept of making changes too quickly is that you cannot learn a new language in one day. So why would you think you could change your eating and exercise habits that you have had for the majority of your life in one day?

I also asked myself many other questions while developing this program. Here are just a few:

- Why can't I stick with a new program for more than a few weeks and sometimes only a few days?

- What am I thinking and feeling when I decide to buy a new program?

- How do I feel when starting the new program?

- Why do I slip back into my old routine only to put the weight back on quickly?

- How am I going to break this cycle (otherwise known as "yo-yo dieting")?

- How am I going to develop a program that is low cost given our economy, does not require expensive DVD's or monthly product purchases, and can revolutionize the industry?

Through several years of searching, I have found the answers to these questions and have transformed the answers into an innovative program that will revolutionize the industry as we know it. For me personally, the main reason I could not stick with a health program for the long term was my strong cravings for "real food" (bagels, cheese-

burgers, pizza, etc.). My body would go into a shock-like state, sending

strong, painful signals throughout my body that the changes I made

were too drastic. I would then easily find an excuse to cheat on the

diet and convince myself that the diet was unrealistic and that I was

normal to want real food. If you are reading this book, there is a good

chance that you have also failed at other diet programs and can relate

to the pain of strong cravings. Yet whenever I ask someone why he or

she failed to stick with a program long term, the typical answers are

related to many other things: work, not enough time to plan and pre-

pare meals, got tired of the food choices, etc.

Many of us also purchase programs in a disappointed or frustrated

state of mind. Marketers capitalize on this and use this as one of mech-

anisms to influence you to purchase the program. Marketers also do

a great job convincing you that you can look like the person in the ad

in a short period of time. After making the purchase we then have

inspiration and hope believing that "this is the one that is going to work, once and for all." After following the program and achieving

short-term success, we slip back into our old routines and quickly put

the weight back on. The cycle of this experience is summarized below:

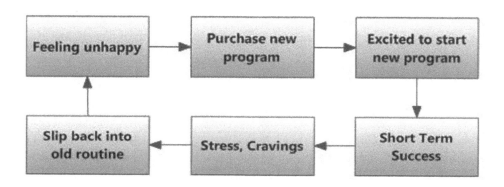

The program I developed is designed to break this cycle. It is designed

for people who need a flexible approach to transforming their minds and

bodies. The program's foundation is based on introducing changes to

your diet and exercise in a controlled manner over a period of time that is

realistic for achieving long-term success. It assumes people will continue

to keep the same routine and favorite eating places and can leverage read-

ing and modern technology (Internet and calorie apps) to educate them-

selves on calorie values of foods. It also assumes that people like different types of foods, will make changes at different rates, and will need to enjoy the foods they love as part of the program.

I would also like to share what this program is *not* about. The program will not transform your body in sixty to ninety days. If you are looking to do that, I encourage you to try a sixty- to ninety-day transformation program, and I sincerely wish you success. In the approximately 80 percent chance you fail in the long term, then pick this book up again and give it a chance to transform your mind and body for long-term success. I also want to be very clear that I do have respect for portions of diet and health programs on the market now. I have learned a great deal about calories, metabolism, nutrition, and exercise. For every program that I have truly followed, I have lost weight. They all share a universal truth: you must burn more calories than you consume. My program also shares this universal truth; however, it takes an innovative approach by factoring in human behavior for changing your dietary and exercise habits for the long term.

# CHAPTER 2

# PROGRAM OVERVIEW

I have named this program "Change Control Diet" because the program is all about controlling the rate at which you make changes to your eating and exercise habits. The term "Change Control" by itself is a term commonly used in the pharmaceutical industry. It is a process to control any changes in order to preserve the safety, efficacy and purity of medicines. I realize the name "Change Control Diet" may be awkward for some; however, I wanted a name for this program that articulated the true essence of this diet. I also wanted to stay away from a "marketing gimmick name"; this has been a huge frustration of mine with the weight loss industry. To help visualize this concept of controlling the rate of change, let's say John is consuming on average 4200 calories per day prior to starting this program. Here is how a standard diet will implement changes to John's caloric intake and meal choices over time:

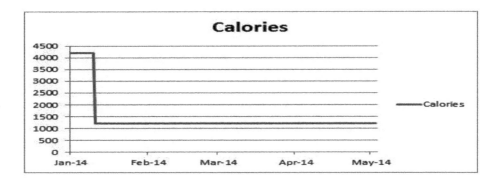

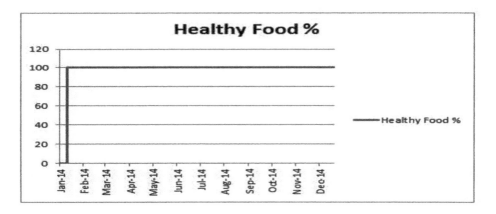

As you can see from these graphs, the rate of change is very intense for standard diets, going from one extreme to the other in only one day. The Change Control Diet is different; it's all about controlling the rate of change. Here is an example of how changes are introduced to

John's calories and food choices following the Change Control Diet:

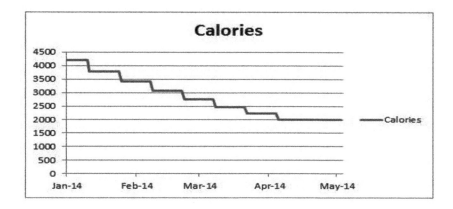

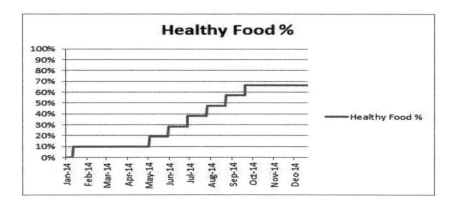

As you can see from these graphs, the Change Control Diet

controls the rate of change in a progressive stepwise manner which allows your body the proper time to adjust to changes. The program consists of seven levels of dietary changes and five levels of exercise changes to your routine. You progress through the levels at your own pace, only moving to the next level after your body adjusts to the changes in the previous level of the program. The levels are focused on weekly goals, not daily goals. For example, there are seven days in a week, which equates to a total of twenty-one meals and twenty-one snacks per week (eating a total of six times per day). It is much easier to set a weekly goal versus a daily goal to allow flexibility for unexpected events, changes to your schedule, stress, etc. One of the key reasons for my failures at other diets was finding an excuse to quit an entire program based on one bad day at work. Focusing on the week versus the day was an amazing mindset alteration for me.

The food portion of the program is captured in the table below:

## Change Control Diet Food Levels

| Level | % Change in Food Choices from Start | Per Week Real Meals | Per Week Healthy Meals | Per Week Real Snacks | Per Week Healthy Snacks |
|---|---|---|---|---|---|
| 1 | 9.5 | 19 | 2 | 19 | 2 |
| 2 | 19.0 | 17 | 4 | 17 | 4 |
| 3 | 28.5 | 15 | 6 | 15 | 6 |
| 4 | 38.0 | 13 | 8 | 13 | 8 |
| 5 | 47.5 | 11 | 10 | 11 | 10 |
| 6 | 57.0 | 9 | 12 | 9 | 12 |
| 7 | 66.5 | 7 | 14 | 7 | 14 |

"Real Meals" and "Real Snacks" are the foods you are currently eating. For me this is cheeseburgers, pizza, potato chips, chocolate chip cookies, etc. You can also think of "Real Meals and Snacks" as "Choice Meals and Snacks", you are choosing what you want to eat. "Healthy Meals" and "Healthy Snacks" are the foods your doctor recommends for you to eat: grilled chicken, grilled fish, fruits, vegetables, whole-wheat grains, etc. Healthy meals and snacks are also real food as well (e.g. it is not imaginary food); however, my naming convention here is based on changing negative associations. I do not feel guilty eating cheeseburgers and pepperoni pizza; I love this type of food and grew up on it. In following standard diets previously, I always had a sense of guilt when I cheated. I realized during the development of this program that it was completely ridiculous to feel guilty eating something I enjoyed.

Now here is the amazing part: You will start losing weight at Level One of this program. Level One makes a small change in your dietary choices and reduces your daily calories in 10 percent weekly increments to minimize the pain from cravings. The key to losing weight is eating smaller portions six times a day to jump start your metabolism. You don't have to change your food choices to reduce calories. You just need to cut down on the portions, eat six times a day, and educate yourself on calories. Prior to this program, I typically used to eat only two meals a day. I would skip breakfast, eat a reasonable lunch in front of coworkers, and eat a very large dinner when home. Eating only twice a day significantly slowed down my metabolism. The slower your metabolism, the fewer calories

you burn and the more fat that gets stored on your body.

The exercise portion of the program takes a similar approach to

introducing changes in a controlled manner and is represented in the

table below:

### Change Control Diet Exercise Levels

| Level | Exercise Sessions Per Week | "I Believe" Positive Thinking Daily |
|---|---|---|
| 1 | 2 Times Low Intensity 30 Minutes | 5 Minutes a.m. |
| 2 | 3 Times Low Intensity 30 Minutes | 5 Minutes a.m. |
| 3 | 3 Times Moderate Intensity 30 Minutes | 5 Minutes a.m. |
| 4 | 3 Times Moderate Intensity 45 Minutes | 5 Minutes a.m. |
| 5 | 3 Times High Intensity 45 Minutes | 5 Minutes a.m. |

From an exercise perspective, this program assumes you are not currently exercising regularly. Through many years of my own trial and error, I have found that starting an exercise program at a low intensity level (e.g., fat burning zone) is better than jumping right into an intense workout regime. Taking this approach will help reduce strong cravings for food after working out. In my own experience, I have gone from being a "coach potato" to exercising for several sixty-minute, high-intensity sessions a week, only to "binge eat" at night on the days of my intense workouts. While still providing a cardiovascular benefit from the exercise, this approach defeats the purpose when you are trying to lose weight because you will end up consuming all of the calories you burned off at night.

The exercise portion of the program is also optional depending on your current health and schedule demands. I highly recommend that everyone exercise; however, we need to be realistic in that not everyone is physically able to exercise, and some people have very demanding schedules. The exercise portion of the program is also designed to run parallel to the food portion of the program; however, matching levels of the food program with the exercise program is not required. For example, you may progress through multiple levels of the food program while choosing to stay at Level One of the exercise program. The opposite is also true: you may spend several months at Level One of the food program but be able to progress through Level Three of the exercise program during those months. The table below lists scenarios and includes comments to assist with illustrating this aspect:

| Scenario | Description | Example of Level progression |
|----------|-------------|------------------------------|
| 1 | Jim is a 25-year-old obese male who eats frequently through-out the day and is consuming 10,000 calories per day prior to starting a program. Jim does not exercise currently. | Jim spends 6 months at Level One of the Food Guidelines due to the number of 10% weekly reductions in calories to obtain the recommended daily calorie value of 2,400 calories. However, Jim is able to progress through Level Four of exercising during this same 6-month period because as he loses weight, he has more energy to exercise. |
| 2 | Sarah is a 52-year-old female who is con-suming 1,700 calories daily but only eats twice a day. Sarah works two jobs to support her family and does not have time to exercise. | Sarah spends 3 weeks at Level One of the Food Program because she only needed to reduce calories by ~6% to achieve the recommended 1,600 calories per day. Sarah takes 3 weeks to adjust to eating 6 times a day. Sarah then progresses through the remaining Food Levels and spends an average of 2 weeks at each level. Sarah does not set additional time aside to exercise given her long work day and family commitments; however, she frequently takes the stairs and adds extra physical activity to her normal routine. |
| 3 | Juan is a 14-year-old boy who is a line-man on the school football team but is 50 pounds over-weight and has a high amount of body fat. Juan is currently consuming on aver-age 8,500 calories per day. From an exercise perspective, Juan has practice 4 days a week and a game every Friday. | Juan spends 4 months at Level One of the food program due to the number of 10% weekly reductions in calories to obtain the recommended daily calorie value 2,800–3,200 calories per day given his very active exercise schedule with football. Given Juan's practice and game schedule, he is starting this program already at an advanced level of exercise. During the off-season of football, Juan will progress through additional levels of the food program while maintaining Level Five of the exercise program. |

# CHAPTER 3

# POSITIVE THINKING AND CORE BELIEFS

Let us start with a simple definition of positive thinking. Positive thinking is believing in a positive outcome to a situation. As it applies to this program, positive thinking is believing in yourself: Believe that you can make small changes to your diet and exercise habits over time. Start off every day with the two words "I Believe" and say them to yourself several times throughout the day and night. Spend at least five minutes every morning focusing your thoughts on how you want to look at the end of this program and what specific choices you are going to make today to help you achieve that goal. While this may sound ridiculous to some people, let me ask you a question: do you think anyone who has made a significant change in her life or a significant contribution to the world told herself every morning that she was going to fail? I am known by friends and coworkers as an optimist. However, I was not born an optimist; I made the choice to be one. Everyone has the ability and power from within to change. It all starts with you believing in yourself.

There are five core beliefs of the Change Control Diet:

**#1 – Standard diet programs fail for most people because they introduce changes to the diet too quickly.** This results in your body going into a "shock-like state" in that you have very strong cravings for the food you are used to eating. Changes to your eating and exercise habits will be more successful long term if they are introduced in a controlled manner over a period of time rather than as a radical change on day one of a program. Your weight-loss goal per week should range from 0.5 pounds to 2 pounds maximum.

**#2 – There is a universal truth to losing weight: you must burn more calories than you consume.** This universal truth should be applied on a weekly basis, not a daily basis. The reason for a weekly mindset versus a daily mindset is to allow flexibility with stresses and cravings. Everyone cheats on a diet and has a bad day once in a while. This program factors in this reality, with the goal of changing people's association that diets are too restrictive.

**#3 – Take ownership and accountability for your own food choices and exercise habits.** Diet programs on market are too restrictive and prescriptive—they tell you how to shop (e.g., grocery list), exactly what to eat, and how to exercise. The Change Control Diet is different. While the focus is on introducing changes in a controlled manner, it has you take ownership in planning your own meals and exercise program. You are smart enough to plan calorie values for meals and still enjoy the foods you love. From an exercise perspective, the most important thing is to adjust your schedule to make the time to exercise. Stop making excuses that you don't have time and find a way to make time to exercise. Keep it simple—you do not need a special exercise program and/or expensive equipment to lose weight. You simply need to burn more calories than you consume. View exercise as a tool to help you burn more calories. It's that simple.

**#4 – Say "I believe" to yourself every morning.** The power of a positive mind is the key to long-term success. Do not use guilt or negative emotion as your motivator. True, there are many success stories from people who have used negative emotion as a motivator, but that typically means they hit "rock bottom"—they had let themselves get to a point where they were very unhappy with their image, and/or their health was very poor. I have tried to use negative emotion myself as a motivator and was able to achieve short-term success, but I would always fall hard and end up even heavier than when I started. If you happen to be going through a very challenging, "rock-bottom" part of your life now, the best thing you can do is to use positive thoughts and energy to help you get through this period of your life. Leverage the love and support of people who care about you. If you have negative people in your life who always bring you down, consider making some changes.

**#5 – Focus on changing your habits slowly; the results will follow.** The goal of this program is to change your food and exercise habits for the long term in a controlled manner. As mentioned previously, factor losing 0.5–2 pounds per week at the most. Do not live by the scale or the "tale of the tape." It is highly recommended that you weigh yourself only once a week and measure inches of your body areas that you're focusing on once a month. Do not get discouraged if you do not lose weight in a week; what this is telling you is that you need to consume fewer calories for your meals and/or you need to increase your exercise level. I have had weeks on this program where I did not lose weight, but I was also weight lifting and adding muscle to my body. I have also had a few weeks where I deviated from the program and consumed more calories than I burned due to stress. Here was the key to my long-term success: I focused on changing my habits when dealing with stress versus how I was going to lose the weight.

# CHAPTER 4

# Understanding and Estimating Calories

For this program, think of calories as energy. Your body needs energy to function properly. Energy for your body comes from two sources: the food you eat and the stored fat on your body. Consuming more calories than your body needs in a day results in your body storing excess energy as fat. Burn more calories than you consume and your body burns the fat stored on your body, which results in you losing weight and inches. Another way to visualize this is to view your body as an engine. Your engine runs constantly to allow for moving, breathing, heart beating, etc. To keep the engine burning and using fuel from both tanks (consumed food and stored fat) throughout the day, you need to eat smaller portions six times a day.

This program requires you to understand and estimate calorie values of foods; however, you are not required to track every calorie every day. Instead, you establish calorie goals for meals and snacks. For example, if your daily calorie goal is 2,000 calories and you need to eat six times, then you can break down your calorie goals as follows:

| Meal | Calories |
|------|----------|
| Breakfast | ~500 |
| Midmorning Snack | ~200 |
| Lunch | ~500 |
| Midafternoon Snack | ~200 |
| Dinner | ~500 |
| Evening Snack | ~100 |
| Total | ~2000 |

Now, before we dive into calorie tables, I would like to share an example of how your current food choices can be used to achieve this goal. Your normal breakfast is an egg sandwich with two eggs, a sausage patty, and a hash brown, which totals ~700 calories. Instead of making a drastic change on day one of this program, try this instead: eat half the meal for breakfast (~350 calories) and the other half three hours later for your midmorning snack. This approach will still reach your morning calorie total of ~700 calories. This program also places a huge focus on "approximately" (~). If you're like most people, you will drive yourself crazy if you try to accurately track every single calorie every day. I tried tracking every calorie for a week and drove myself to a high level of frustration, and I realized that this approach would fail with most people. For the Change Control Diet, the most important aspects of the food program are being able to estimate calories, reduce your portions to achieve your calorie goals, and eat six times a day. Another important aspect is that this program recognizes that different people have different preferences and personality profiles. My personality profile is someone who prefers flexibility and variety, and I love being spontaneous. If you are a person who prefers control and schedules, you may want to consider tracking your calories daily. For example, my wife falls into this category and prefers to track calories using a free app she found on her iPhone. The choice is up to you.

To start educating yourself on food calories, go through your house and make a table of common foods and calorie values that are in your house. Here's an example of some of the items in my house:

| Food | Amount | Calories |
|---|---|---|
| Thomas English Muffin | 1 muffin | 100 |
| Thomas Cinnamon Raison Muffin | 1 Muffin | 140 |
| White Bread | 1 Slice | 80 |
| Jewish Rye Bread | 1 Slice | 90 |
| Whole Wheat Bread | 1 Slice | 60 |
| Eggs | 1 egg | 80 |
| Egg Whites | 1 serving, 3 tbsp. | 25 |
| Cheese, Muenster | 1 slice, 21grams | 80 |
| Cheese, American | 1 slice, 21grams | 70 |
| Cheese, Cheddar | 1/4 cup, 28 grams | 110 |
| Lunch Meat, Roast Beef | 2 oz., 56 grams | 70 |
| Lunch Meat, Ham | 2 oz., 56 grams | 60 |
| Butter | 1 tbsp. | 100 |
| Peanut Butter | 2 tbsp., 32 grams | 190 |
| Strawberry Preserves Jelly | 1 tbsp., 20 grams | 50 |
| Frozen Waffles | 2 waffles, 70 grams | 190 |
| Frozen Cinnamon Waffles | 2 waffles, 76 grams | 250 |
| Frozen Pancakes | 3 pancakes, 105 grams | 250 |

| Food | Amount | Calories |
|------|--------|----------|
| Frozen Breakfast Sausage | 2 patties, 45 grams | 150 |
| Shoprite pineapple fruit cup | 1 cup | 70 |
| Cheetos | 28 grams, 21 pieces | 150 |
| Potato Chips | 28 grams, 11 chips | 160 |
| Pretzel Rods | 30 grams, 3 pretzel rods | 120 |
| Buggles (Snack) | 30 grams, 1/3 cup | 160 |
| Drumstick (Ice Cream) | 1 Drumstick | 190 |

The amazing part of this for me was learning that a simple peanut butter and jelly sandwich can easily be 500–600 calories if you load on the peanut butter (three tablespoons) and jelly (three tablespoons). Adding butter to a 100-calorie English muffin can also easily add 50 calories (butter ~100 calories per tablespoon).

Second, use the Internet and free calorie apps to further educate yourself on caloric values for the foods you commonly eat. For example, the United States Department of agriculture has a website at ndb.nal.usda. gov that lists over 8,000 food items. This database is free to the public and is searchable. A slice of pizza with regular crust and no additional toppings in this database is 285 calories. A slice of pizza with regular crust and sausage topping is 325 calories. Instead of this book listing numerous tables of food items, you will educate yourself more quickly by getting this information yourself for the foods you commonly eat.

Also, if you are eating at fast-food chains, they now have food calorie values on the menus. Unfortunately, it took an act of Congress to get fast-food chains to post the caloric values on the menus (passed in 2010, implemented in 2011). For example, there are several varieties of the Egg McMuffin sandwich from McDonalds:

- Egg White Egg McMuffin – 250 calories

- Egg McMuffin – 300 calories

- Sausage McMuffin – 370 calories

- Sausage McMuffin With Egg – 450 calories

Now, by having an Egg White Egg McMuffin sandwich of 250 calories versus a Sausage McMuffin with Egg sandwich of 450 calories, you can reduce your breakfast calories by 200 calories with one simple choice change. Also, when I do have McDonalds, regardless of whether it is for breakfast, lunch, or dinner, I typically avoid the hash browns, French fries, and drinks with calories to help me stay within a caloric goal for a meal.

Once you understand the calories of the common foods you eat, it's easy to apply this understanding to restaurants and "on the go" meals. For example, eating a quarter-pound cheeseburger at a restaurant is going to be anywhere between 500 and 700 calories on average, depending how much cheese and other toppings go on the burger. If you have a strong craving for a cheeseburger, go ahead and order it. Just reduce the amount of toppings and replace the French fries with steamed vegetables. In addition, drink water in place of a beverage with calories. Making these modifications can reduce the calorie count of your meal by approximately 400–700 calories. Another strategy—in the event you are craving French fries and a beer to go with your cheeseburger—is to eat half the meal and save the leftovers for lunch or dinner the following day. I found this strategy to work better than following other diets that required me to order a turkey burger or grilled chicken sandwich in place of the cheeseburger. Remember, the key to start losing weight is to simply focus on reducing calories at each meal, not to drastically change your choices.

Liquid calories and condiments are also important to keep track of, and these calories do count as part of your daily caloric and meal goals. For example, here are some caloric values of beverages and condiments in my house:

| Beverage/ Condiment | Amount | Calories |
|---|---|---|
| Fat-Free Milk | 1 cup, 240 mL | 90 |
| Orange Juice | 1 cup, 240 mL | 110 |
| Coffee Creamer, Chocolate Carmel | 1 tbsp. | 35 |
| Coffee Creamer, Vanilla Carmel Sugar Free | 1 tbsp. | 15 |
| Coffee Creamer, Caramel Macchiato | 1 tbsp. | 35 |
| Coke | 1 can, 355 mL | 140 |
| Root Beer | 1 can, 355 mL | 170 |
| Diet Soda (coke, ginger ale, sprite) | 1 can, 355 mL | 0 |

| Water | any size | 0 |
|---|---|---|
| Snapple Orangeade | 1 bottle, 473 mL | 190 |
| Chocolate Syrup | 2 tbsp. | 100 |
| Ketchup | 1 tbsp. | 20 |
| Dijon Mustard, Spicy Mustard | 1 tbsp. | 5 |
| Light Mayonnaise | 1 tbsp. | 35 |

As I mentioned previously, this program does not require you to count every calorie, but you do need to educate yourself on calories to achieve your caloric goals for meals. For example, I put about two tablespoons of chocolate caramel coffee creamer in my coffee every day. I am adding approximately seventy calories to my coffee, and these seventy calories are also loaded with sugar. Instead of putting a strict restriction on low sugar, I simply count the calories as part of my breakfast calorie total.

Now that we have covered the food and beverage side of calories, it is equally important to understand how exercise helps to burn calories. While your body is constantly burning calories to function, your metabolism will burn more calories if you exercise. It does not matter when you exercise (morning versus afternoon versus evening); what matters is that you make the time to exercise. This can also be as simple as parking farther from work, taking the stairs throughout the day, etc. While the number of calories you burn depends on your weight and heart rate, here is a table (on pages 40-41) of exercise calorie values for thirty minutes of activity from Nutribase.com:[6]

The last aspect of calories is understanding the calorie deficit required to lose one pound in a week. Note here that I am stating a calorie deficit because you can accomplish this through eating less or exercising more, or a combination of both. The National Institutes of Health (NIH) does a nice job explaining this aspect: "There is no magic formula for weight loss. You must eat fewer calories than you burn. Just how many calories you burn daily depends on factors such as your body size and how physically active you are. If you have to lose weight, it's important to do so slowly. Aim for losing no more

6  http://www.nutribase.com/exercala.htm (The NutriBase Exercise Calories Expenditures Chart)

than ½ pound to 2 pounds a week. One pound equals 3,500 calories.

So, to lose 1 pound a week, you need to eat 500 calories a day less or

burn 500 calories a day more than you usually do."[7]

---

7  http://www.nhlbi.nih.gov/hbp/prevent/h_weight/c_lose.htm (National Institutes of
Health, National Heart, Lung and Blood Institute, How can I lose Weight?)

| Activity (30 Minutes) | 120 lbs. | 130 lbs. | 140 lbs. | 150 lbs. | 160 lbs. | 170 lbs. | 180 lbs. | 190 lbs. | 200 lbs. | 220 lbs. | 240 lbs. | 260 lbs. | 280 lbs. | 300 lbs. |
|---|---|---|---|---|---|---|---|---|---|---|---|---|---|---|
| Aerobic dancing (low impact) | 138 | 149 | 161 | 172 | 184 | 195 | 207 | 218 | 230 | 253 | 276 | 299 | 322 | 345 |
| Aerobics step training, 4" step (beginner) | 174 | 189 | 203 | 218 | 232 | 247 | 261 | 276 | 290 | 319 | 348 | 377 | 406 | 435 |
| Aerobics, slide training (basic) | 180 | 195 | 210 | 225 | 240 | 255 | 270 | 285 | 300 | 330 | 360 | 390 | 420 | 450 |
| Basketball (game) | 264 | 286 | 308 | 330 | 352 | 374 | 396 | 418 | 440 | 484 | 528 | 572 | 616 | 660 |
| Basketball (leisurely, nongame) | 156 | 169 | 182 | 195 | 208 | 221 | 234 | 247 | 260 | 286 | 312 | 338 | 364 | 390 |
| Bicycling, 10 mph (6 minutes/mile) | 150 | 162 | 175 | 188 | 200 | 213 | 225 | 237 | 250 | 275 | 300 | 325 | 350 | 375 |
| Bicycling, 13 mph (4.6 minutes/mile) | 240 | 260 | 280 | 300 | 320 | 340 | 360 | 380 | 400 | 440 | 480 | 520 | 560 | 600 |
| Housework | 108 | 117 | 126 | 135 | 144 | 153 | 162 | 171 | 180 | 198 | 216 | 234 | 252 | 270 |
| Jogging, 5 mph (12 minutes/mile) | 222 | 240 | 259 | 278 | 296 | 315 | 333 | 352 | 370 | 407 | 444 | 481 | 518 | 555 |
| Jogging, 6 mph (10 minutes/mile) | 276 | 299 | 322 | 345 | 368 | 391 | 414 | 437 | 460 | 506 | 552 | 598 | 644 | 690 |
| Running, 08 mph (7.5 minutes/mile) | 366 | 396 | 427 | 458 | 488 | 518 | 549 | 579 | 610 | 671 | 732 | 793 | 854 | 915 |
| Running, 09 mph (6.7 minutes/mile) | 396 | 429 | 462 | 495 | 528 | 561 | 594 | 627 | 660 | 726 | 792 | 858 | 924 | 990 |
| Running, 10 mph (6 minutes/mile) | 420 | 455 | 490 | 525 | 560 | 595 | 630 | 665 | 700 | 770 | 840 | 910 | 980 | 1050 |
| Snow shoveling | 234 | 253 | 273 | 292 | 312 | 332 | 351 | 371 | 390 | 429 | 468 | 507 | 546 | 585 |
| Soccer | 234 | 253 | 273 | 292 | 312 | 332 | 351 | 371 | 390 | 429 | 468 | 507 | 546 | 585 |

| Activity (30 Minutes) | 120 lbs. | 130 lbs. | 140 lbs. | 150 lbs. | 160 lbs. | 170 lbs. | 180 lbs. | 190 lbs. | 200 lbs. | 220 lbs. | 240 lbs. | 260 lbs. | 280 lbs. | 300 lbs. |
|---|---|---|---|---|---|---|---|---|---|---|---|---|---|---|
| Stair climber machine | 192 | 208 | 224 | 240 | 256 | 272 | 288 | 304 | 320 | 352 | 384 | 416 | 448 | 480 |
| Stair climbing | 168 | 182 | 196 | 210 | 224 | 238 | 252 | 266 | 280 | 308 | 336 | 364 | 392 | 420 |
| Swimming (25 yards/minute) | 144 | 156 | 168 | 180 | 192 | 204 | 216 | 228 | 240 | 264 | 288 | 312 | 336 | 360 |
| Swimming (50 yards/minute) | 270 | 292 | 315 | 338 | 360 | 382 | 405 | 428 | 450 | 495 | 540 | 585 | 630 | 675 |
| Table Tennis | 108 | 117 | 126 | 135 | 144 | 153 | 162 | 171 | 180 | 198 | 216 | 234 | 252 | 270 |
| Tennis | 192 | 208 | 224 | 240 | 256 | 272 | 288 | 304 | 320 | 352 | 384 | 416 | 448 | 480 |
| Trimming hedges | 126 | 136 | 147 | 158 | 168 | 178 | 189 | 199 | 210 | 231 | 252 | 273 | 294 | 315 |
| Vacuuming | 90 | 98 | 105 | 112 | 120 | 128 | 135 | 142 | 150 | 165 | 180 | 195 | 210 | 225 |
| Walking, 2 mph (30 minutes/mile) | 72 | 78 | 84 | 90 | 96 | 102 | 108 | 114 | 120 | 132 | 144 | 156 | 168 | 180 |
| Walking, 3 mph (20 minutes/mile) | 96 | 104 | 112 | 120 | 128 | 136 | 144 | 152 | 160 | 176 | 192 | 208 | 224 | 240 |
| Walking, 4 mph (15 minutes/mile) | 120 | 130 | 140 | 150 | 160 | 170 | 180 | 190 | 200 | 220 | 240 | 260 | 280 | 300 |
| Weight training (40 sec. between sets) | 306 | 332 | 357 | 382 | 408 | 433 | 459 | 484 | 510 | 561 | 612 | 663 | 714 | 765 |
| Weight training (60 sec. between sets) | 228 | 247 | 266 | 285 | 304 | 323 | 342 | 361 | 380 | 418 | 456 | 494 | 532 | 570 |
| Weight training (90 sec. between sets) | 150 | 162 | 175 | 188 | 200 | 213 | 225 | 237 | 250 | 275 | 300 | 325 | 350 | 375 |

For those people who need to lose a lot of weight, you need to set realistic expectations on how long this will take you to achieve your goal weight. The below table will help you with setting realistic goals for the timing to reach your goal weight:

| Number of Pounds to Lose | Number of Weeks to Reach Your Goal Weight | | | |
|---|---|---|---|---|
| | 1/2 pound per week | 1 pound per week | 1.5 pounds per week | 2 pounds per week |
| 10 | 20 | 10 | 7 | 5 |
| 25 | 50 | 25 | 17 | 12.5 |
| 50 | 100 | 50 | 33 | 25 |
| 75 | 150 | 75 | 50 | 37.5 |
| 100 | 200 | 100 | 67 | 50 |
| 150 | 300 | 150 | 100 | 75 |
| 200 | 400 | 200 | 133 | 100 |

Now, here's the issue with doing a sixty- to ninety-day transformation program and the *Biggest Loser* reality show: people are losing weight too quickly, easily five to fifteen pounds per week, depending on the person. This is not a successful strategy for the long term and is why 80 percent of Americans put the weight back on after stopping a diet. Now, for the people who have taken this approach and have kept the weight off long term, I am sincerely happy for you. I am not looking for a debate with the doctors and trainers of these programs. I am, however, looking to help the approximately 1.4 billion people in the world for whom this approach will not work. It's time for a change and a new direction in the industry.

# CHAPTER 5

# FOOD AND CALORIE GUIDELINES

Before we cover the food and calorie guidelines, I want to stress a few key points based on feedback from my family and friends following this program:

- You should spend one to two weeks educating yourself on calories for your routine and then stop counting calories. Let's face it; everyone follows a routine, even when it comes to food. And as you progress through the levels, once you have your routine down at each level, stop counting calories, portion control will come naturally.

- There is a calorie formula in this chapter to establish calorie goals for meals and snacks. **You can make changes to this formula to fit your routine as long as your approximate total calories are achieved.** For me, I am a forty one year old male that should consume ~2200 calories on the days I am not exercising. I don't care if I end up consuming 2053 or 2407 calories, it does not matter in the grand scheme of things. Think of this program as a journey to change your habits for long term success, not as a program that requires you to go crazy with calorie counting and following something exactly.

- From a women's perspective (thank you Kristen and Kelly), it is very important to avoid going to extremes to look good for a special event (a wedding, reunion, party, etc.). I too have struggled with this in the past. I always wanted to look good for the beach and started each New Year off with an aggressive diet and exercise regimen. It would always end up with me back in my old routine by March and me wearing a T-shirt on the beach. The other key aspect for women applies during "that time of the month" where I am extra nice to my wife. My wife typically gains weight during this week because of extra fluid retention and she also goes to a lower level of the Food Program to allow more "real food" throughout the week. Again, this program is about a journey and the big picture. It's not about obsessing over every bite.

The food guidelines are summarized below:

- The most important aspect of the food guidelines is eating smaller portions six times a day. This approach will increase your metabolism and enable your body to burn more fat.
- For eating six times a day, try to eat within the first hour of waking up in the morning and spacing at least two hours between your meals and snacks. So for example, if you wake up at 6:00 a.m. every day:

- Breakfast – 7:00 a.m.

- Midmorning Snack –10:00 a.m.

- Lunch –12:00 p.m.

- Midafternoon Snack – 3:00 p.m.

- Dinner – 6:00 p.m.

- Evening Snack – 8:00 p.m.

- Initially, it is more important to focus on calories versus setting numerous rules on what you can't eat. This is why Level One of the program only requires you to eat two healthy meals and two healthy snacks per week. And this is good from a cost perspective because you keep the food that is currently in your house.

- Drink several glasses of water throughout the morning, day, and evening to stay hydrated. Minimize soda, sweet drinks, and diet drinks. While diet soda has zero calories, it has the potential to cause cravings for other sugary items.

- Spend a minimum of seven days at each food level in the program. It is perfectly acceptable to spend several weeks at a level in the program. Keep your focus on changing your eating habits slowly, not on how fast you can progress through each level. Remember, your goal is not to run a marathon tomorrow.

While I was developing this program, my wife came to me one day and said, "I have no idea how you are losing so much weight; you eat constantly and are still eating junk food." The reason is that I decided that after many years of failing on other diets that instructed me exactly what to eat, I was going to just focus on calorie goals for meals and snacks instead. The Change Control Diet focuses on a set of general guidelines and common sense. For example, from a common-sense perspective, you do not need a book or doctor to tell you that a quarter pound beef cheeseburger with four strips of bacon is not good for you. In addition,

I believe that life is too short to deprive yourself of foods you enjoy. This is why I designed the highest level of this program to still be able to enjoy seven "real meals" and seven "real snacks" per week. The reason my wife did not realize I was dieting was that during the workweek, she would only see me eat in the evenings. What she did not see was that while I was at Level Seven of the food program, I would eat healthy meals and snacks in the mornings and afternoons, and I saved my "real meal" and "real snack" for the evening. The other benefit of this approach was avoiding inconveniencing my wife in planning for dinners. Most people who plan and prepare meals in the household can relate to running out of ideas for dinner. Add the complexity of one family member being on a strict diet, and that's a recipe for extra hassles with meal planning.

As stated previously, the most important aspect of the food guidelines is eating smaller portions six times a day to speed up your metabolism. Metabolism, as defined by the dictionary at

Merriam-Webster.com, is the "sum of all the chemical reactions that take place in every cell of a living organism, providing energy for the processes of life and synthesizing new cellular material."[8] Here's the amazing part that some people may not be aware of: you actually burn calories eating and digesting food. Similarly to the "think of your body as an engine" analogy, you can also think of your metabolism as an engine that runs everything. The more frequently you eat (staying within calorie goals) and move throughout the day, the more calories you will burn. My wife has previously lost approximately twenty pounds very quickly on another popular meal plan diet that had her eating six times a day. But there was a huge problem with following this long term: my wife was only consuming on average 1,000–1,200 calories per day following this program, and she was frequently starving. This is because she was consuming 400–600 fewer calories than what she should have been consuming. When my

---

8  http://www.merriam-webster.com/dictionary/metabolism (Merriam-Webster Dictionary, Metabolism *Concise Encyclopedia* Definition)

wife got tired of the food plan and stopped the program, she quickly

put the twenty pounds back on.

As a general guideline for how many calories you should have

daily, here is a table that was developed by the National Institutes of

Health (NIH). It contains recommended daily calories by age, gender,

and activity level:

| Gender | Age (years) | Activity Level | | |
|---|---|---|---|---|
| | | Sedentary | Moderately Active | Active |
| Female | 4–8 | 1,200 | 1,400–1,600 | 1,400–1,800 |
| Female | 9–13 | 1,600 | 1,600–2,000 | 1,800–2,000 |
| Female | 14–18 | 1,800 | 2,000 | 2,400 |
| Female | 19–30 | 2,000 | 2,000–2,200 | 2,400 |
| Female | 31–50 | 1,800 | 2,000 | 2,200 |
| Female | 51+ | 1,600 | 1,800 | 2,000–2,200 |
| Male | 4–8 | 1,400 | 1,400–1,600 | 1,600–2,000 |
| Male | 9–13 | 1,800 | 1,800–2,200 | 2,000–2,600 |
| Male | 14–18 | 2,200 | 2,400–2,800 | 2,800–3,200 |
| Male | 19–30 | 2,400 | 2,600–2,800 | 3,000 |
| Male | 31–50 | 2,200 | 2,400–2,600 | 2,800–3,000 |
| Male | 51+ | 2,000 | 2,200–2,400 | 2,400–2,800 |

As defined by the NIH,

a.  Sedentary means a lifestyle that includes only the light physical activity associated with typical day-to-day life.

b.  Moderately active means a lifestyle that includes physical activity equivalent to walking about 1.5 to 3 miles per day at 3 to 4 miles per hour, in addition to the light physical activity associated with typical day-to-day life.

c.  Active means a lifestyle that includes physical activity equivalent to walking more than 3 miles per day at 3 to 4 miles per hour, in addition to the light physical activity associated with typical day-to-day life.[9]

This table does not factor in your current weight, your current metabolism, how much muscle is on your body, or how many calories you are currently consuming daily (prior to starting this program).

9  http://www.nhlbi.nih.gov/health/public/heart/obesity/wecan/healthy-weight-basics/balance.htm (National Institutes of Health, National Heart, Lung and Blood Institute, Balance Food and Activity)

For Level One of the program, it is recommended that you do not reduce your daily caloric intake by more than 10 percent at a time and that you eat six times a day. For example, if you are a thirty-five-year-old obese male who is currently consuming 5,000 calories a day, dropping to 2,200 calories a day in one day will shock your system, and you have approximately an 80 percent chance you will fail long term. Instead, this program has you reducing your daily total calories by 10 percent initially and spreading this over eating six times a day. This would result in 4,500 calories a day for starting off on day one at the first level of this program. More is explained about this approach in Chapter 8 – Food Level One.

The following table represents a recommended daily caloric plan for the Change Control Diet after you determine your daily caloric total:

| Daily Calories | Breakfast | Midmorning Snack | Lunch | Mid-afternoon Snack | Dinner | Evening Snack |
|---|---|---|---|---|---|---|
| 1,200 | 300 | 120 | 300 | 120 | 300 | 60 |
| 1,300 | 325 | 130 | 325 | 130 | 325 | 65 |
| 1,400 | 350 | 140 | 350 | 140 | 350 | 70 |
| 1,500 | 375 | 150 | 375 | 150 | 375 | 75 |
| 1,600 | 400 | 160 | 400 | 160 | 400 | 80 |
| 1,700 | 425 | 170 | 425 | 170 | 425 | 85 |
| 1,800 | 450 | 180 | 450 | 180 | 450 | 90 |
| 1,900 | 475 | 190 | 475 | 190 | 475 | 95 |
| 2,000 | 500 | 200 | 500 | 200 | 500 | 100 |
| 2,100 | 525 | 210 | 525 | 210 | 525 | 105 |
| 2,200 | 550 | 220 | 550 | 220 | 550 | 110 |
| 2,300 | 575 | 230 | 575 | 230 | 575 | 115 |
| 2,400 | 600 | 240 | 600 | 240 | 600 | 120 |
| 2,500 | 625 | 250 | 625 | 250 | 625 | 125 |
| 2,600 | 650 | 260 | 650 | 260 | 650 | 130 |
| 2,700 | 675 | 270 | 675 | 270 | 675 | 135 |
| 2,800 | 700 | 280 | 700 | 280 | 700 | 140 |
| 2,900 | 725 | 290 | 725 | 290 | 725 | 145 |
| 3,000 | 750 | 300 | 750 | 300 | 750 | 150 |
| 3,100 | 775 | 310 | 775 | 310 | 775 | 155 |
| 3,200 | 800 | 320 | 800 | 320 | 800 | 160 |

For caloric goals not listed in this table, the formulation is:

- Breakfast, Lunch, Dinner – 75 percent of your total daily calories (25 percent at each meal)

- Midmorning Snack and Midafternoon Snack – 20 percent of your total daily calories (10 percent at each snack)

- Evening Snack – 5 percent of your total daily calories

So for the example of the thirty-five-year-old obese male who is consuming 5,000 calories prior to starting this program:

- 0.9 x 5,000 calories = 4,500 calories total per day to start this program

- Breakfast, Lunch, Dinner – 4,500 calories x 0.25 = 1,125 calories per meal

- Midmorning and Midafternoon snacks – 4,500 calories x 0.1 = 450 calories per snack

- Evening Snack – 4,500 x 0.05 = 225 calories

I have experimented with different caloric values for meals and snacks. You can make modifications to this based on your schedule and energy demands, but it is important not to go significantly over or under your calories for the day. For example, if you have a physical job and need to consume more calories earlier in the day to keep you going, that is fine; just use common sense. For me, on the days when I exercise in the evenings, I eat smaller meals and snacks at the beginning of the day and larger snacks and meals later in the day to ensure I have energy to support my evening workouts. Alternatively, for days when I work out in the mornings, I eat a larger breakfast and midmorning snack.

Your meals should be balanced with protein and carbohydrates—do not have a protein-only meal or a carbohydrate-only meal. "Real meals" and "real snacks" are the foods you normally eat. "Healthy meals" and "healthy snacks" are the foods your doctor recommends for you to eat: grilled chicken, grilled fish, fruits, vegetables, whole grains, etc.

The below table contains examples of real foods and healthy food alternatives for this program. On the notion of keeping it simple, this program is not about becoming a health-food nut. It's about finding the right balance between real food and healthy food to help you achieve your weight-loss and health goals.

| Change Control Diet Food Category | Real Foods | Healthy Foods Alternatives |
|---|---|---|
| Animal Proteins | Prime Rib, Delmonico Steak, T-Bone Steak, Roast Beef, Cheeseburger, Meatballs, Sausage, Fried Chicken, Bacon, etc. | Lean Steak (Sirloin), Salmon, Flounder, Shrimp, Lobster, Grilled/Baked Chicken, Turkey, Turkey Burger, Turkey Meatballs, etc. |
| Dairy | Whole Milk, Yogurt, Cheese, Ice Cream, etc. | Fat-Free Milk, Fat-Free Yogurt, Low-Fat Cheese, etc. |
| Bread/Pasta (Complex Carbohydrates) | White Bread, White Pasta, White Rice, Baked Potatoes, etc. | Whole Grain Bread, Whole Wheat Bread, Whole Wheat Pasta, Brown Rice, Oatmeal, Yams, etc. |
| High-Sugar Snacks (Simple Carbohydrates) | Skittles, Butterfingers, Snickers, Starburst, Sherbet, Candy, Cookies, Chocolate Cake, etc. | Fresh Fruits: Oranges, Grapefruits, Apples, Pears, Plums, Strawberries, Blueberries, etc. |

| Change Control Diet Food Category | Real Foods | Healthy Foods Alternatives |
|---|---|---|
| Crunchy Snacks | Bagged Processed Salty Snacks: Potato Chips, Pretzels, Cheetos, etc. | Carrots, Celery, Peppers, Cucumbers, etc. |

Here are some general themes to eating healthier that should not be a surprise to anyone:

- Replace red meat with grilled chicken, turkey, or fish

- Replace fried food with a baked alternative—for example, panko-breaded baked chicken versus fried chicken

- Replace crunchy processed snacks (potato chips, pretzels, etc.) with a crunchy vegetable (carrots, peppers, celery, etc.)

- Replace sugary processed snacks (cookies, candy, etc.) with fruit (oranges, apples, grapes, etc.)

- For on-the-go meals and fast food, choose low-calorie options: grilled chicken versus a burger, don't order the fries, etc.

Work with your doctor to establish additional guidelines if necessary for your current health and weight-loss goals. Remember, the key to this diet is eating fewer calories more frequently throughout the day. Only a 9.5 percent change is required in food choices for Level One of the program, which equates to two healthy meals and two healthy snacks per week at Level One of the program. You will start losing weight at Level One of the program because your metabolism will increase by eating smaller portions six times a day.

The last section of the Food Guidelines covers proper hydration. According to the NIH, "although there is no research to identify the exact amount of water you should drink, experts usually recommend drinking six to eight eight-ounce glasses of water daily."[10] Water is essential to life. Our bodies are made of approximately two-thirds water, and you will die in a few days without drinking water.

---

10   http://www.nlm.nih.gov/medlineplus/ency/article/002471.htm (National Institutes of Health, Medline Plus, Water in Diet, August 2011)

Another benefit of drinking water throughout the day is to help with cravings. Sometimes our bodies send signals that we interpret as being hungry when in fact your body is signaling that it needs more water.

# CHAPTER 6

# EXERCISE GUIDELINES

I highly encourage everyone to exercise. However, you can lose weight without exercising on this program, and as a result, the exercise portion of this program is optional. There are several reasons why I made this optional:

- I don't want people to use it as an excuse to not follow my program. Simply put, some people do not enjoy exercise. If you fall into this category, I recommend that, after losing some weight initially through following the food portion of this program, you find a type of exercise you enjoy.
- Some people are physically unable to exercise.

- Some people have very demanding schedules and do not have time to exercise.

The issue with not exercising is that you are doing your metabolism and cardiovascular system a disservice. If you don't have time to set aside in your day for exercise, then incorporate exercise into your day by parking farther away from work, taking the stairs versus the elevator, getting up and moving around several times a day if you have an office job, etc. If you take your kids to a sports practice, instead of sitting and watching, go for a walk around the field. The key is to move more than you currently do in your normal routine. I would also challenge you to take away from technology time (texting, Facebook, Twitter, etc.) to find the time to exercise.

The exercise guidelines are simple and are summarized below:

- Exercise is anything that gets you moving outside of your normal routine currently.

- Make sure when you exercise that your heart rate is elevated to either a low-intensity or high-intensity zone. You can purchase a heart-rate monitor or check your heart rate by measuring your pulse on the inside of your wrist. Count how many pulses you feel in fifteen seconds and multiply this number by four to get your heart rate.

- Start off slowly with exercise. Keep it simple by using walking as your starting exercise for this program. There is no need to overcomplicate it by requiring you to purchase exercise DVDs for three payments of $39.95, to join a gym, etc. If you enjoy exercise DVDs and/or joining a gym, go for it. My wife, for example, is what I call an "exercise DVD fanatic." You have to do what works for you.

- Spend a minimum of one week at each level. The goal is to increase time and intensity over time to allow your body to adjust to exercise and reduce the amount of strong cravings for food that are triggered by exercising.

As I previously mentioned, changes to your exercise schedule are introduced in a controlled manner. Remember, the goal is not to run a marathon tomorrow; it is to change your exercise habits over the long term. The exercise levels of the program were covered in Chapter 2 – Program Overview and are listed here again:

## Change Control Diet Exercise Levels

| Level | Exercise Sessions Per Week | "I Believe" Positive Thinking Daily |
|---|---|---|
| 1 | 2 Days Low Intensity 30 Minutes | 5 Minutes a.m. |
| 2 | 3 Days Low Intensity 30 Minutes | 5 Minutes a.m. |
| 3 | 3 Days Moderate Intensity 30 Minutes | 5 Minutes a.m. |
| 4 | 3 Days Moderate Intensity 45 Minutes | 5 Minutes a.m. |
| 5 | 3 Days High Intensity 45 Minutes | 5 Minutes a.m. |

Low intensity for this program is defined as having your heart rate between 50 percent and 69 percent of your maximum heart rate. Walking for thirty minutes is a great way to start for exercising at low intensity. High intensity is when your heart rate is between 70 percent and 85 percent of your maximum heart rate. This includes running and circuit training with weights. Moderate intensity for this program is when, for at least half your work out, you are in the high-intensity heart range. For example, Level Three is thirty minutes of moderate-intensity exercise three days a week. This means that for each thirty-minute exercise session, you have your heart rate in high intensity for at least fifteen minutes. The table below lists low-intensity and high-intensity heart ranges by age:

| Age | Maximum Heart Rate | Low-Intensity Heart Rate Range (50%-69% of Max Heart Rate) | | High-Intensity Heart Rate Range (70%-85% of Max Heart Rate) | |
|---|---|---|---|---|---|
| 5 | 215 | 108 | 148 | 151 | 183 |
| 10 | 210 | 105 | 145 | 147 | 179 |
| 15 | 205 | 103 | 141 | 144 | 174 |
| 20 | 200 | 100 | 138 | 140 | 170 |
| 25 | 195 | 98 | 135 | 137 | 166 |
| 30 | 190 | 95 | 131 | 133 | 162 |
| 35 | 185 | 93 | 128 | 130 | 157 |
| 40 | 180 | 90 | 124 | 126 | 153 |
| 45 | 175 | 88 | 121 | 123 | 149 |
| 50 | 170 | 85 | 117 | 119 | 145 |
| 55 | 165 | 83 | 114 | 116 | 140 |
| 60 | 160 | 80 | 110 | 112 | 136 |
| 65 | 155 | 78 | 107 | 109 | 132 |
| 70 | 150 | 75 | 104 | 105 | 128 |
| 75 | 145 | 73 | 100 | 102 | 123 |

There is some debate in the industry of fat-burning zone (low intensity) versus cardio zone (high intensity) and which one is best. In the fat-burning (low-intensity) zone, 50 percent of the calories are burned from fat. In the cardio (high-intensity) zone, 40 percent of calories are burned from fat. The Change Control Diet does not place a huge emphasis on the difference between these; the most important aspect is to get moving to burn calories. Common sense will tell you that you will burn more calories at a high-intensity heart rate versus a low-intensity heart rate for the same period of time exercising. Your focus should be on progressing through the levels below at a comfortable pace, allowing a minimum of seven days at each level.

For monitoring your heart rate, I recommend purchasing a heart-rate monitor that has a strap for your chest and a monitor watch for your wrist. Most monitors also track the number of calories you burn when you exercise. If you cannot afford to purchase a heart-rate monitor, you can check your heart rate manually as previously described and can still use the table above as a guideline for low-intensity and high-intensity heart rate workouts.

Before, during, and after your workout, you need to make sure you are drinking plenty of water. I typically drink a glass of water right before exercising and another glass during exercise. Staying hydrated is very important because it helps remove toxins and reduce chances of injury (muscle strains, tears, etc.).

Stretching is equally important. You should spend a few minutes stretching prior to exercising and then after exercising. I never believed in stretching after exercising until I pulled a calf muscle running. Since I have been stretching both before and after exercising, I have avoided injury.

# CHAPTER 7

# ESTABLISHING A BASELINE AND RELEASING NEGATIVE ENERGY

Before starting this program, you must have a good understanding of your current eating and exercise habits as well as how many calories on average you are consuming daily. Take one week without changing anything in your dietary choices, and record the following each day:

- The times of your meals, snacks, and beverages. List what you eat and drink and estimate the calorie values you are consuming (remember, liquid beverages and condiments count). It is important to also count how much water you are currently drinking in a day—part of this program requires several glasses of water each day.

- Your feelings each day, paying special attention to whether stress triggers consuming more calories.

- Your surroundings and environment. Do you always eat in certain areas of your house? For example, I was able to stop snacking late nights by working on the second floor of my house because the first floor contained my food cabinets and refrigerator. Do you "cave in" when driving past fast-food restaurants on your way home from work? These are the types of things you should be observing during the week.

- Your family and friends are equally important. Are you surrounded by positive people? Is there anyone in your life now who has a negative impact or is not supportive? The watch-out here is that negative people can also influence your failures. You need to either be able to not let others' negativity impact you, or you need to make some changes to minimize your interactions with negative people in your life.

After seven days, calculate the average daily calories you consume in one day (add up the calories of seven days and divide that number by seven). This value will be used later in Level One of the food program.

If you have not met with your doctor recently for a general checkup (physical), I would recommend that you do so to get a physical and general blood work. If you are overweight or obese, there may be other health risks that will need to be monitored, including high blood pressure, high cholesterol, and diabetes. I had both high blood pressure and high cholesterol prior to starting this program. Unfortunately high blood pressure and high cholesterol run in my family, so I had to go on medication. My doctor was pleased with my weight-loss progress, though, and I was able to avoid going on higher doses of blood-pressure medicine and cholesterol medicine by losing weight, exercising, and making better food choices.

Before starting the program, it is very important to release negative energy by letting go of all your past failures in losing weight. If you meditate normally, you can accomplish this through meditation. If you do not meditate regularly, I recommend the following approach: on a piece of paper, make a list of all the reasons you think you have failed at previous diets over the years. Write down each diet name, approximately how long you were able to follow it, and why you stopped it. Common reasons include not enough time, too much work, too many family commitments and responsibilities, too hard to follow, too expensive, etc. Now here's the fun part: take several deep breaths and/or listen to music to put you in a relaxed mood. Now rip this piece of paper up into at least twenty pieces. As you rip the paper, take several deep breaths and let go of your past failures. After you are done, place the pieces of paper in a paper-recycling bin, take another deep breath, and say to yourself, "I believe," and think of how you want to look at the end of this program.

# CHAPTER 8

# FOOD LEVEL ONE

Food Level One is by far the most important level of this program. You may spend one week at this level, or you may spend several months. It really depends on your current daily calories, how many times you are eating in a day currently, your metabolism, and how well your body responds to changes. Remember, this is the key reason for failing at other diets: the other diets shocked your system by giving you a "one-size-fits-all" menu to follow with no accounting whatsoever of where you are starting from. An analogy here would be someone you never met sending you an email asking you to buy him a new outfit. The obvious challenge is that you never met him and do not know his clothing size or his style preferences. How do you think that would work out? I would say similar to industry weight-loss failure statistics in the United States—you have at least an 80 percent chance of failing.

Pick a day of the week that is ideal for starting this program, and conduct your weigh-in and body-tape measurements of your body areas that you want to lose inches from (for example, stomach, chest, and buttocks). I recommend avoiding Mondays as a starting day. For example, I started this program on a Friday to allow four days after the weekend to burn off any excess calories that I may have consumed on the weekend. Remember, this program is about achieving long-term, life-changing results; it is not about making ridiculous sacrifices on the weekends. Enjoy the party on the weekend (in moderation); life is too short. For weigh-in it is very important to weigh yourself and take your measurements first thing in the morning after using the bathroom. For the night before, it is also important to avoid a high-sodium dinner and high-sodium snacks. Sodium increases water retention, and you will weigh more than usual. The worst meal I have consumed the night before weigh-in is Chinese food, which is generally very high in sodium (read the sodium content of a soy sauce bottle label as a reference point). In addition, water weighs a lot, so I would not recommend exercising the night before weigh-in because you will consume extra water during your workout that may not be excreted prior to weigh in. It is OK to exercise in the morning or afternoon the day before weigh-in.

Select your target daily calories from the NIH table previously covered in Chapter 5, which is also listed here again for convenience:[11]

| Gender | Age (years) | Activity Level | | |
|---|---|---|---|---|
| | | Sedentary | Moderately Active | Active |
| Female | 4–8 | 1,200 | 1,400–1,600 | 1,400–1,800 |
| Female | 9–13 | 1,600 | 1,600–2,000 | 1,800–2,000 |
| Female | 14–18 | 1,800 | 2,000 | 2,400 |
| Female | 19–30 | 2,000 | 2,000–2,200 | 2,400 |
| Female | 31–50 | 1,800 | 2,000 | 2,200 |

11  http://www.nhlbi.nih.gov/health/public/heart/obesity/wecan/healthy-weight-basics/balance.htm (National Institutes of Health, National Heart, Lung and Blood Institute, Balance Food and Activity)

| Female | 51+ | 1,600 | 1,800 | 2,000–2,200 |
| --- | --- | --- | --- | --- |
| Male | 4–8 | 1,400 | 1,400–1,600 | 1,600–2,000 |
| Male | 9–13 | 1,800 | 1,800–2,200 | 2,000–2,600 |
| Male | 14–18 | 2,200 | 2,400–2,800 | 2,800–3,200 |
| Male | 19–30 | 2,400 | 2,600–2,800 | 3,000 |
| Male | 31–50 | 2,200 | 2,400–2,600 | 2,800–3,000 |
| Male | 51+ | 2,000 | 2,200–2,400 | 2,400–2,800 |

From Chapter 7, you determined how many calories on average you are consuming daily. It is very important to identify the difference of the NIH recommendation and the number of calories you are currently consuming. Just as we want to introduce healthy foods in a controlled manner to your diet, we also need to reduce your current calories in a controlled manner. The program requires that you will not reduce your calories by more than 10 percent at a time. So for example, if you are a thirty-five-year-old female at a low activity level, your daily target caloric value from the table above is 1,800 calories. However, if you are currently consuming on average 3,000 calories a day, you would start off on the first day of this diet with a 2,700 calorie daily goal. An easy way to calculate a 10 percent reduction in calories is to take your current daily calories and multiply it by 0.9 (so in this case 3,000 calories x 0.9 = 2,700 calories). If you do not follow this approach of reducing your calories in 10 percent increments, you have a high probability of failing. For example, going from 3,000 calories a day to 1,800 calories in one day is a 40 percent reduction in calories. Your chances of strong cravings and discomfort will greatly increase with this drastic reduction in calories.

For each reduction in calories, spend a minimum of seven days (one week) at the calorie level. You are ready to reduce calories a further 10 percent if you achieved staying within your daily caloric goal for a minimum of six days out of the week. This allows for one "bad day" in the week in the event you are not able to stay within your daily caloric goal on all seven days. Please note, I am not promoting that you should have one day of binge eating. I am promoting that you should not give up on a diet just because you had one bad day. This program is also designed to change your association that diets are too restrictive. If you really think about it, the first week of this program only requires a 10 percent reduction in calories and a 9.5 percent change in food choices (two healthy meals and two healthy snacks) throughout the week. This is a goal that can be achieved easily if you put your mind to it.

You then continue with weekly 10 percent reductions at Level One until you hit your recommended daily caloric intake from the National Institute for Health Table. The table below contains examples of the number of calorie reductions necessary to reach a 2,000 calorie per day goal:

| Current Daily Calories | First Adjustment | Second Adjustment | Third Adjustment | Fourth Adjustment | Fifth Adjustment | Total Adjustments to reach ~ 2,000 Calories per day |
|---|---|---|---|---|---|---|
| 30,000 | 27,000 | 24,300 | 21,870 | 19,683 | 17,715 | 26 |
| 25,000 | 22,500 | 20,250 | 18,225 | 16,403 | 14,762 | 24 |
| 20,000 | 18,000 | 16,200 | 14,580 | 13,122 | 11,810 | 22 |

| 15,000 | 13,500 | 12,150 | 10,935 | 9,842 | 8,857 | 19 |
|--------|--------|--------|--------|-------|-------|-----|
| 10,000 | 9,000 | 8,100 | 7,290 | 6,561 | 5,905 | 15 |
| 5,000 | 4,500 | 4,050 | 3,645 | 3,281 | 2,952 | 9 |
| 4,000 | 3,600 | 3,240 | 2,916 | 2,624 | 2,362 | 7 |
| 3,000 | 2,700 | 2,430 | 2,187 | 1,968 | NA | 4 |

In summary, Food Level One requires you to make weekly 10 percent calorie reductions until you reach your NIH recommended calorie value. During the weekly calorie reductions you are required to eat six times a day and have two healthy meals and two healthy snacks during the week. Once you have completed all of your weekly calorie reductions and achieve six out of seven days at the NIH recommended daily calorie value, you are ready for Food Level Two.

# CHAPTER 9

# FOOD LEVELS TWO THROUGH SEVEN

The food levels are captured again below for convenience:

## Change Control Diet Food Levels

| Level | % Change in Food Choices from Start | Per Week Real Meals | Per Week Healthy Meals | Per Week Real Snacks | Per Week Healthy Snacks |
|-------|-------------------------------------|---------------------|------------------------|----------------------|-------------------------|
| 1 | 9.5 | 19 | 2 | 19 | 2 |
| 2 | 19.0 | 17 | 4 | 17 | 4 |
| 3 | 28.5 | 15 | 6 | 15 | 6 |
| 4 | 38.0 | 13 | 8 | 13 | 8 |
| 5 | 47.5 | 11 | 10 | 11 | 10 |
| 6 | 57.0 | 9 | 12 | 9 | 12 |
| 7 | 66.5 | 7 | 14 | 7 | 14 |

Upon successful completion of Food Level One, you are ready for Level Two. Level Two involves replacing an additional two "real meals and snacks" with two "healthy meals and snacks" throughout the week. While this is a 19 percent change in food choices before starting this program, it is only 9.5 percent change from Level One of the program. The key aspect from a mindset perspective is to focus on the latter; e.g., "I am only making a 9.5 percent change in my food choices by having two more healthy meals and snacks." Spend a minimum of one full week at Food Level Two. Success at Food Level Two is defined as:

- Consuming four healthy meals and four healthy snacks throughout the week

- Eating six times a day for a minimum of six days

- Staying at your recommended total NIH daily calorie value for a minimum of six days

An important note is that if you are exercising as well, you may experience additional cravings for food. It is acceptable to increase your daily caloric total as defined in the recommended NIH caloric value table listed in Chapter 5 – Food and Calorie Guidelines to account for exercise days. However, remember the goal here is to burn more calories than you consume to lose weight, so if you are fine staying at the lower "Sedentary" level of calories and can manage cravings, then I would recommend staying at this level of calories. For me personally, it depends on how hard I work out. If I work out at low intensity, I can stay at the sedentary caloric value; however, if I have a moderate- or high-intensity workout, I do need to consume extra calories that day.

For progressing through the remaining Food Levels of the program, you spend a minimum of seven days at each level. You are ready to move to the next level of the program if you:

- Consume the defined amount of healthy meals and healthy snacks for the level throughout the week

- Eat six times a day for a minimum of six days

- Stay within your daily recommended NIH calorie value for a minimum of six days

From a goal perspective, the goal of this program is to find the right balance of real food and healthy food that will allow you to achieve your weight-loss and health goals. The goal of this program is **NOT** to:

- Race through the levels as quickly as you can to obtain Level Seven. Racing through the levels will most likely result in failure for the long term. In addition to the success criteria to progress to the next level, you should leverage your intuition (e.g., what feels right to you).

- Stay at Level Seven for the rest of your life. In fact, you may not even need to achieve Level Seven if you find a level in which you and your doctor determine that you are healthy (you achieved your weight-loss goal, your cholesterol is fine, your blood work is good, etc.).

As with Level One of this program, each level may require you to spend several weeks there before progressing to the next level. As mentioned above, if you reach your weight-loss and health goals prior to reaching Level Seven and you and your doctor are satisfied with your health, you can stay at that level. For me personally, I progressed to Level Seven and stayed at this level for several months to help with reducing my cholesterol. However, I get tested for cholesterol regularly and am able to live at Level Five or Six of this program (depends on the week), which means I eat healthy approximately 50 to 60 percent of the time. The key for following this program for life is practicality—it has to work for you and be easy to follow. What better than a program that allows you to achieve your weight-loss and health goals and still enjoy the foods you love throughout the week?

As part of "practicality," the other aspect is that you are obviously going to enjoy your vacations. While you are on vacation, here are the guidelines to follow:

- To heck with counting food calories, enjoy your vacation!

- Do try to keep to the spirit of this program by eating smaller portions six times a day versus three big meals a day if you can. If you can't, that's OK. Smile—you are on vacation!

- And last but not least, never count liquid calories on vacation—that's why they call it vacation!

So obviously my sense of humor is coming through here, but I am serious: enjoy your vacations. This is what they are for. You do need to keep your commitment to this program for when you return from vacation by picking up at the same level prior to leaving for vacation. One week will not create significant challenges adjusting quickly back to the level you were at before vacation. In addition, I have found that because of this program, I am much better behaved on vacations because my stomach is significantly smaller and holds less food now. My eating and exercise habits have also changed permanently—they are part of my daily routine and require minimal effort to follow.

# CHAPTER 10

# EXERCISE LEVELS ONE THROUGH FIVE

The exercise levels are captured again below for convenience:

### Change Control Diet Exercise Levels

| Level | Exercise Sessions Per Week | "I Believe" Positive Thinking Daily |
|-------|----------------------------|-------------------------------------|
| 1 | 2 Days Low Intensity 30 Minutes | 5 Minutes a.m. |
| 2 | 3 Days Low Intensity 30 Minutes | 5 Minutes a.m. |
| 3 | 3 Days Moderate Intensity 30 Minutes | 5 Minutes a.m. |
| 4 | 3 Days Moderate Intensity 45 Minutes | 5 Minutes a.m. |
| 5 | 3 Days High Intensity 45 Minutes | 5 Minutes a.m. |

I encourage you to reread Chapter 6 – Exercise Guidelines. Here is a condensed version of the guidelines:

- Exercise is anything that gets you moving outside of your current normal routine.
- Make sure to monitor your heart rate to ensure you are achieving the proper intensity of your exercise level.
- Start off slow with exercise and keep it simple.
- Spend a minimum of one week at each level.

As mentioned previously, when you exercise your body may require additional calories to minimize cravings. Do not go above the NIH recommended value for the days you exercise. For example, if you are a twenty-year-old female, the NIH recommended calorie values are:

- Sedentary (no exercise) – 2,000 calories
- Moderately Active – 2,000–2,200 calories

- Active – 2,400 calories

In Chapter 5 – Food and Calorie Guidelines, we covered the definitions of sedentary, moderately active, and active provided by NIH. As they relate to this program, here are the guidelines for increasing calories on the days you exercise:

**Increasing Calorie Values for Exercise Days**

| Level | Exercise Sessions Per Week | Calorie Recommendation for the Day You Exercise |
|---|---|---|
| 1 | 2 Days Low Intensity 30 Minutes | Sedentary* |
| 2 | 3 Days Low Intensity 30 Minutes | Sedentary* |
| 3 | 3 Days Moderate Intensity 30 Minutes | Moderately Active |
| 4 | 3 Days Moderate Intensity 45 Minutes | Moderately Active |
| 5 | 3 Days High Intensity 45 Minutes | Active |

*For Levels One and Two, the NIH would most likely rate this level of exercise as moderately active because the definition of moderately active is walking 1.5–3 miles per day at three to four miles an hour. So if it is necessary to increase calories for you at Level One and Two, that is perfectly acceptable. I am recommending trying not to initially because the goal is to burn more calories than you consume. When I exercise at low-intensity levels, I do not have additional calorie cravings however, everyone is different and you need to do what works for you.

Some may ask, why exercise if I have to consume more calories? The primary reasons are that exercise offers cardiovascular benefits, increases your metabolism, and reduces stress. For me, exercise is therapeutic at relieving stress. I joke with my friends and family and define it as therapy for me; e.g., "I had a therapy session this morning, so I am very relaxed today."

How long you stay at each level really depends on your fitness prior to starting this program—your age, your health, etc. As with the food guidelines, this program is not about racing to get to Exercise Level Five or staying at Level Five for your entire life. Find what works for you and feels right.

Also, the exercise program does not have an 80/20 rule built into the exercise program levels. Since this only calls for two to three days a week and thirty to forty-five minutes of exercising each day, you must meet all criteria for that week to progress to the next level. However, similar to vacation guidelines for the food levels, you can determine your exercise guidelines for vacations.

# CHAPTER 11

# EVERYONE CHEATS—THE 80/20 RULE

Everyone cheats on diets—it's a fact (or at least it's a fact for the hundreds of millions of people who have failed at diets previously). This is why the Change Control Diet factors this reality into the program. Even on the highest food level of this program, you can have one piece of chocolate cake every day (adjusting the portion size to stay within your calorie goal for snacks, of course). And even if you have one bad day where you violate a few rules, this program considers the week a success, and you can move forward to the next level in the program. I built this aspect into the program because our bodies are not designed for 100 percent perfection.

In corporate America I am a big fan of the 80/20 rule. My definition of the 80/20 rule is this: as long as we are 80 percent confident in our decisions and assumptions, let's move forward. Otherwise we lose days, weeks, or months—and sometimes we fail entire projects—by striving for 100 percent perfection. This is easier said than done depending on how your brain is wired. For people who are comfortable with ambiguity (the unknown), this is easy. For the majority of people I work with, though, moving forward at 80 percent confidence is an uncomfortable feeling. I have the same experience outside of work as well: a large percentage of friends and family strive for the "100 percent perfection" and prefer to do things in an orderly fashion.

Here's the problem with the 100 percent perfection goal for classical diets: we get cravings when we see, smell, or hear about the foods and beverages we love. Our brains send signals to our bodies on how much we are going to enjoy consuming the item, and it is very hard to turn these signals off. And for me personally, whenever I would cheat on another diet I would use this as a reason to quit the entire program. I would say to myself, "Well, I cheated, so I can't follow this diet anymore." But in reality my body was really saying, "Hey, buddy, this program is horrible; what were you thinking by cutting my calories by so much on day one of the program!"

The key to successfully using the 80/20 rule is repetition. It also helps if within your "positive sphere of influence" (Chapter 17 – Change the Game) you have someone who is creative and comfortable with ambiguity. In my career, I have had to coach staff and team members on changing their thought process to adjust to this approach by letting them know that it is OK to make mistakes. When you follow the 80/20 rule, you also have a 20 percent chance that you made a wrong assumption that will result in a mistake. So this will not work if you tell someone to follow the 80/20 rule and then reprimand them when a mistake happens—you need to walk the talk. So here is a program that is telling you that it is OK to have one bad day in the week. As mentioned previously, I am not promoting that you should do this on purpose, I am simply accounting for the fact that our bodies are not designed for 100 percent perfection.

Taking this thinking one step further, it is possible to have a bad week or several bad weeks due to life's challenges. During the year 2013, in which I finalized this program and this book, I had the following events occur:

- My wife slipped on ice and broke her shoulder.

- My wife had emergency back surgery for a blown disc to avoid permanent nerve damage in her leg and foot.

- My wife and daughter were in a car accident and hit a deer (they were fine, thank god, but our vehicle had several thousand dollars' worth of damage).

- I partially slipped a disc in my back doing a labor-intensive yard project and spent a few months in physical therapy to resolve the problem.

- My wife's aunt passed away unexpectedly from a short battle with lung cancer.

You can't control what life throws at you, but you can control how you respond. Sure, I have had weeks on this program when I was not able to follow the program exactly. However, I did not use it as a reason to quit the program. In fact, I did just the opposite: I made this program even stronger by calling this out as a fact of life and modifying the highest level of my program to allow you to either have one "real meal" and "real snack" per day or to save these up for a fun weekend. As we say in the United States, shit happens! I am sure I will have future weeks where life's challenges will not allow me to follow this program. However, I am confident that I will follow it for the rest of my life nonetheless. Eating smaller portions six times a day is now my daily routine.

So in the unfortunate event that you have a life challenge thrown at you, remember this chapter. You are in control of how you respond to life's challenges. It is OK to make mistakes; our bodies are not designed for 100 percent perfection.

# CHAPTER 12

# TRACKING PROGRESS

As mentioned in Chapter 8 – Food Level One, pick an optimal day of the week to start this program. For the typical work habits and lifestyle of the average American, I recommend starting this diet on a Friday to allow a few days after the weekend to burn off any excess calories that may have been consumed. I also recommend creating a table with the following columns to track your progress:

| Week | Date | Weight | Stomach Circumference | Chest Circumference | Thighs/Buttocks Circumference |
|---|---|---|---|---|---|

Remember the following key points for weigh in:

- Weigh yourself once a week. Put the scale in your closet or another room so that you are not weighing yourself daily. If you historically weighed yourself every day, this is a tough change. The rationale for doing this is to help create more focus on changing your eating and exercise habits versus reacting to a number on the scale daily.

- Measure the circumference of the fat storage areas on your body using a body measuring tape once every four weeks. I found some inconsistencies when measuring myself weekly and believe that this is due to how much water is in your body and variability due to differences in how you measure. It is important to measure in the same place for each area and to use the same amount of tension when using the body measure tape.

- Weigh and measure yourself in the mornings after you use the bathroom initially in the morning (e.g., within ten minutes of waking up).

- Do not eat high sodium (salty) foods the day or night before weigh-in (high sodium makes you retain more water).

- Do not exercise the evening before weigh-in because if you are exercising properly, you will be consuming several glasses of water during your workout. Note: it is acceptable to exercise the day before; just do so in the morning or afternoon.

As the weeks go by, you will start to see results. It is important to not get discouraged if you do not lose weight every week on this program. Below is a table of my actual results for the 2013 year:

| Week | Date | Weight lbs. | Stomach | Chest | Total Weight Loss | Total Inches Lost Stomach | Total Inches Lost Chest |
|---|---|---|---|---|---|---|---|
| Start | 1/4/2013 | 225.3 | 46.25 | 46.50 | Start | Start | Start |
| 4 | 2/1/2013 | 220.4 | 45.13 | 46.19 | 4.9 | 1.13 | 0.31 |
| 8 | 3/4/2013 | 211.4 | 42.00 | 44.63 | 13.9 | 4.25 | 1.87 |
| 12 | 4/1/2013 | 209.4 | 41.50 | 44.00 | 15.9 | 4.75 | 2.50 |
| 16 | 4/26/2013 | 206.0 | 40.75 | 43.63 | 19.3 | 5.25 | 2.75 |
| 20 | 5/24/2013 | 206.0 | 41.00 | 43.75 | 19.3 | 5.25 | 2.75 |
| 24 | 6/21/2013 | 205.0 | 40.50 | 43.25 | 20.3 | 5.75 | 3.25 |
| 28 | 7/19/2013 | 209.0 | 41.25 | 44.00 | 16.3 | 5.00 | 2.50 |
| 32 | 8/16/2013 | 208.0 | 41.00 | 44.00 | 17.3 | 5.25 | 2.50 |

| 36 | 9/13/2013 | 207.6 | 41.00 | 44.00 | 17.7 | 5.25 | 2.50 |
| 40 | 10/11/2013 | 206.2 | 40.50 | 42.75 | 19.1 | 5.75 | 3.75 |
| 44 | 11/8/2013 | 204.8 | 39.50 | 42.25 | 20.5 | 6.75 | 4.25 |
| 48 | 12/6/2013 | 199.8 | 38.75 | 42.00 | 25.5 | 7.50 | 4.50 |
| 52 | 1/3/2014 | 200.0 | 38.75 | 42.00 | 25.3 | 7.50 | 5.25 |
| 56 | 1/31/2014 | 194.8 | 38.50 | 41.50 | 30.5 | 7.75 | 5.75 |

As I mentioned in the previous chapter, I had a very tough year while finalizing this program and book. I had weeks when not only did I not lose weight, but I actually gained weight. Here is why I am proud to share these results: I am "walking the talk" in the sense that life has challenges, and I decided to stick with the program and not spiral up to 225 pounds again. This program is a transformation journey. It is acceptable to hit some bumps along the way. In addition, I am also very proud of my results: in 56 weeks on this program, I have lost a total of 30.5 pounds, 7.75 inches from my stomach, and 5.75 inches from my chest. The most amazing feeling is that I have not been in the 190s since my early twenties, and I now have twice the energy as I did before starting this program.

# CHAPTER 13

# ADJUSTING CALORIE VALUES AND BREAKING A PLATEAU

It's important to realize that during Food Level One, your body is going to need time to adjust to eating six times a day and to the calorie-reduction steps, in the event you are starting from a higher baseline calorie value compared to the NIH recommendation. As a result, you may not lose weight initially. Remember, the formula for losing weight is a simple universal truth: you must burn more calories than you consume. Before starting this program, you need to factor in whether you were keeping the same weight, gaining weight, etc. Some people, on the other hand, may lose weight more quickly than the recommended 0.5 to 2 pounds per week. My experience has been that the heavier and younger you are, the more quickly you will lose weight.

Before adjusting calorie values, you must successfully complete Food Level One of the program. The rationale for this approach is to keep your focus on staying at the NIH recommended minimum daily calorie value (sedentary level). We need to focus your thoughts and behavior on the idea that eating is good for you and necessary to be healthy. Dropping caloric intake values significantly below the NIH sedentary values is dangerous if followed for the long term. Your body will not get the proper nutrition to remain healthy. I have also watched documentaries on TV about people with eating disorders. I have seen people who consume fewer than 1,000 calories a day and look absolutely horrible. I am sharing this point to remind you that being skinny does not equal being beautiful. I know plenty of people who are overweight, and they are absolutely beautiful. Any diet that changes this beauty is a recipe for disaster.

Remember from Chapter 4 that in order to lose a pound in a week, you need to burn 3,500 calories more than you consume. In the event you have two consecutive weeks in which you did not lose weight, it is acceptable to adjust calorie values. The first strategy for adjusting calories is to keep your total daily calories at the NIH sedentary calorie level and to increase your exercise frequency and/or intensity to burn more calories in the week. Simply adding additional days of walking for thirty minutes can help greatly.

The second strategy for adjusting calorie values, however, is to keep your NIH sedentary recommended calorie value but have more calories in the morning and afternoon. My wife and I have implemented this approach successfully by consuming ~80 percent of our calories by the afternoon snack and then having a fruit smoothie for dinner and a very light evening snack. Again, do not go below your NIH minimum value for daily calories.

When all else fails, under the guidance of your doctor, determine if it is acceptable to go below your NIH minimum value for daily calories. You also may have an underlining health issue that needs to be addressed. I do not recommend staying below the NIH minimum value long term, but you should align with your doctor on the best approach for you. I would also like to call out that many standard diets completely disregard the NIH recommended calorie values and have you significantly below what you should be consuming. Avoid the quick start/rapid weight loss approach at all costs. For example, a very popular trainer has a program which has you consuming 1100 calories a day for the first week of the program, regardless of your current calories prior to starting the program, age and gender. 1100 calories a day is even below the value that the NIH recommends for a four year old girl. In my own experience of radically dropping calories on other programs, I have typically experienced dizziness, headaches, and feeling fatigued. Your safety and health is far more important than losing weight quickly.

# CHAPTER 14

# STRESS AND CRAVINGS

Before we address cravings, we must cover stress as it relates to this program. It is very important to manage stress for two primary reasons:

- Stress can lead to additional cravings.
- Stress emits and attracts negative energy (if you are stressed and having a bad day, it brings other people down as well).

In my life experiences, I have experienced my fair share of stress. I have also learned a great deal from stress. From personal experience, I know that if stress it not managed properly, it wreaks havoc on your body and makes you more prone to sickness and other health issues.

The below table contains strategies for stress management that I have

personally used and found very useful:

## Stress Management Strategies

| Strategy | Comments |
|---|---|
| Life Importance | Focus on the most important thing in your life and ask yourself the following: five years from now, will this issue matter? This is my number-one strategy for dealing with stress. I always think of my wife and children; they are the most important thing to me. When I focus on them, they bring a sense of calm. |
| Accept & Solve | Recognizing that "shit happens," accept the problem and focus on the solution. Dwelling on the issue does not solve anything and only creates more stress. |
| Distract | Think of something else that has nothing to do with what is causing you stress. I use this strategy before important meetings or public presentations. If I feel myself getting nervous and stressed, I think of something very funny or completely off the wall to distract me. |
| Ten-Minute Rule | Learn to let go in ten minutes or less. For example, my boss called me one Friday morning and shared something that boiled my blood three times over. I set a time limit of ten minutes to get over it because I did not want this to ruin my weekend. To calm myself, I had to apply a combination of focusing on my family, accepting the situation, and putting a plan in place to solve the problem. |

| Strategy | Comments |
|---|---|
| Exercise | Exercise is therapeutic. I exercise three times a week. In the event that I have a bad day, I add extra exercise to manage the stress. |
| Meditation | I am a very spiritual person and enjoy meditation in the mornings. Even if it is for only a few minutes, I make sure to have time every morning for this. |

While this program is designed to minimize cravings and the shock to your system from calorie reductions, you most likely will still encounter cravings from time to time; it is perfectly natural. On the notion of positive thinking, the most important aspect for cravings is to focus your thinking on what you can have. So if you are craving chocolate cake but are out of "real snacks" for the week, focus on how you can still eat chocolate cake next week. In fact, if you want to have that piece of chocolate cake next week, you can have it on seven days even at the highest food level of this program, which allows seven real snacks throughout the week. The below table summarizes strategies for dealing with cravings:

## Cravings Strategies

| Strategy | Comments |
| --- | --- |
| Distract | Think of something else that has nothing to do with food. Focus on what you need to do the following day or week. By keeping focus on non-food-related items, it can greatly help reduce cravings. Generally if you can keep your focus on something else for five to ten minutes, the craving goes away. |
| Drink Water | Sometimes when you think you are hungry, your body is actually just thirsty. Drink a glass of water and wait ten minutes. |
| Brush Your Teeth | Brushing your teeth after meals and snacks is a great way to "formally end" the eating session as well as remove the taste of food from your mouth. Leaving food residue in your mouth and teeth can also send triggers to eat more. |
| Substitution | If you are craving crunchy potato chips, replace with a raw vegetable that crunches (carrots, peppers, etc). Likewise, if you are craving something sweet like ice cream, replace with a fruit (strawberries, oranges, etc). |
| Time Flies | My wife and I say this every year: "I can't believe it's Christmas again." Time flies. It feels like two years ago when I brought my daughter home from the hospital after being born. But she is now thirteen, and I have a ten-year-old son. Apply this strategy of "time flies" for the future. For example, instead of saying, "I can't have chocolate cake today; this is horrible," say, "Before I know it, I will be enjoying chocolate cake next week." |

It is not the end of the world if you fail to avoid your craving, keep your focus on the long term and you will succeed. Where you need to be very careful is if your cravings are causing you to binge eat. Then you may want to consider completely eliminating that item from your diet until you find a way to control it. More is explained about this issue in the next chapter.

# CHAPTER 15

# LOVE AND RESPECT YOUR ARCHENEMY

This is an interesting title for a chapter in a diet book. I will also open this chapter up on the note that this topic is very personal for me. However, I am letting my heart and intuition guide me on this one and feel strongly that this is important to share in order to help others. I have an archenemy. I also love my archenemy. Her name is Alcohol. She is absolutely beautiful and comforts me when I need her.

Following the 80/20 rule, Sunday through Friday early evening, I would avoid alcohol. But come Friday night, I would like to enjoy a few drinks. I love alcohol; it tastes great and takes the edge off. It is a great way to wind down from a stressful workweek and celebrate the start of the weekend. Come Saturday night, I would typically have a few drinks in the evening again. The problem with me having a few drinks on Friday and Saturday nights was that alcohol would send signals throughout my body that I was starving. This would result in late-night binge eating. Potato chips, Doritos, pretzels, ice cream, something on the grill—you name it; it was all fair game at night after a few drinks. And think of the calories—drinking is several hundred calories (~150 calories per drink/beer), and then eating "everything in the house" can result in a few-thousand-calorie night. So what happens when you have a few nights a week where you consume more calories than you can burn? You get fat; it's that simple.

I have also watched several documentaries on TV about obesity. I think it's safe to say that other people in this world also have archenemies when it comes to food. It can be chocolate cake, salty crunchy snacks, ice cream, etc. that triggers signals in your body to binge eat. So let's define an archenemy as anything or anyone that triggers you to consume lots of excess calories. The "anything" aspect is simple:

it can be a particular type of food or it can be stress. The "person" aspect is a sensitive subject. If you have a negative person in your life, he or she may trigger you to consume more calories. For example, do you get stressed out by the thought of having to spend several hours with a particular individual? As a result of this stress, do you eat more to comfort yourself? If you answered yes to both of these questions, then that person is the archenemy of your weight-loss efforts. Unfortunately I do not have the answer for how to change a negative person into a positive person. However, I am hoping that by sharing with you how I defeated my archenemy, you can apply a similar approach for finding the solution to yours.

Regarding my archenemy, I want to be clear that I have not yet found a way to enjoy her without consuming lots of calories after. But what I did find was a better way to manage my stress as described in the previous chapter. By exercising, meditating, and focusing my thoughts on what matters the most to me in this life, I am able to go weeks and months without her. In 2013, I was not with her for fifty days, and then again later in the year for over a hundred days. While I missed her in the beginning, through my time away from her, I have realized that I would only like to be with her on special occasions moving forward. And this is my recommendation if you have an archenemy: find alternate ways to manage your stress levels, and if required, take a long break from your archenemy. In closing, my love for my archenemy remains the same, but I have a much higher level of respect for her now.

# CHAPTER 16

# FOCUS ON CHANGING HABITS VS. RESULTS

For all my previous diet failures, I have always been focused on achieving a number on the scale. I will never forget the time that I did a "fad diet" in my late twenties. I dropped approximately forty pounds very quickly in six weeks and flew way past my goal weight by losing a lot more than what I set out to lose initially. At a family birthday party for my daughter, my mother approached my wife in private and asked her if I was on heroin because I looked so bad. My muscle tone was gone, my skin color was different, and my energy level was very low from lack of proper nutrition. If this was not bad enough, my personality changed on this diet as well. I lost something that is very important to me: my sense of humor. I went from being the life of the party to being a buzzkill. So why did I let myself get that way? Because marketers sold me on what I thought I wanted: achieving a low number on the scale quickly. My corporate America experience had also trained my brain for this approach—if you don't hit your results (performance criteria), you typically lose your job.

As mentioned in the introduction, I went on a lot of soul searching into my own previous failures as I was developing this program. During this journey, I realized that it is not the scale that matters; it is your own happiness that matters. I also realized that while I was very happy in life because of my beautiful wife and children, I was very unhappy with how I looked and felt. And then I asked myself a question: what does a number on the scale have to do with how happy I am? The answer was brutally refreshing: absolutely nothing! And then I asked myself another question: how did I get this way? This answer was simple: because I have bad habits when it comes to food and exercise. Then I realized that for me to achieve happiness, I just needed to focus my energy on changing my eating and exercising habits. And that is how the foundation of this program was formed. Developing this program took me several years of trial and error because of the simple fact that we eat every day, so going "cold turkey" is not a successful strategy for a dietary choices. Going "cold turkey" works for some illegal drug addictions because you are not required to do those drugs to live. You are, however, required to eat to live, and this created a complex set of obstacles for me to work through.

As you go through this program, I cannot stress enough that it is more important to focus on changing your eating and exercise habits versus focusing on achieving a number on the scale. This program is about becoming happy with yourself. If you can look in the mirror and truly say to yourself that you are happy with how you look and feel, then you are done with this program. The corresponding weight and body tape measurements are meaningless. Do not let advertisements, television shows, or anything else define happiness for you. You and only you can do that. For example, I have achieved happiness on this program, and I do not have six-pack abs. Nor do I envision myself ever obtaining six-pack abs. On a comical note, I love cheeseburgers and beer way too much and would rather die five years earlier than live in misery eating tofu and drinking water for the rest of my life!

On a serious closing note for this chapter, let your intuition be your guide to defining what your own happiness looks and feels like. And if you have six-pack abs included in your definition, that's fine. The key message here is to make sure that your intuition and your self-awareness guide you on this journey, not a TV personality or show.

# CHAPTER 17

# CHANGE THE GAME

This chapter covers additional strategies for achieving your weight-loss goals. The first concept is creating a sphere of positive energy around you by engaging friends and family on your journey. I chose my wife and children as my positive sphere of energy. I engaged them one day by writing a note of what I would accomplish in the next fifty days. This note included weight-loss goals, not drinking alcohol for fifty days, and finishing three chapters of this book. I signed the note and hung it on the refrigerator one morning without telling them. When I came home from work that day, my thirteen-year-old daughter greeted me by saying, "Dad, you are a dork!!! Do you realize you can just talk to us and not leave formal letters signed on the refrigerator???" We all got a big laugh out of this. But what they did not realize is that I was sick and tired of verbally telling them that "my diet starts Monday," and I needed a new way to state my commitment and engage them on my journey. Because I took this new approach of engaging them, they were influenced and curious about my progress throughout the fifty days. Not only did I accomplish my goals in fifty days, I used this approach again later in the year. Under the guidance of my daughter, though, I decided to modify the formal signed letter route. Instead, I created a four-month daily calendar and taped it to a wall. I brought my children into the room and told them that this time I was going to not drink alcohol for one hundred days and that I would also finish the rest of my book in one hundred days. An "X" would go through the days as they progressed. The rest is history: I submitted my book a month early and went more than one hundred days without alcohol.

The key message here is to engage your family and friends to create a positive support group. If you have family and friends who also need to lose weight, engage them on this journey and make a formal commitment together. Write a letter and have everyone sign it. Make enough copies so they can all bring it home and hang it on their refrigerators. Just remember to keep your commitments focused on following the program and changing eating and exercise habits, not achieving a number on the scale. Exercising with a significant other or friend helps pass the time, especially if you find exercise boring. Having someone to talk to about cravings and challenges is a great support system.

The other aspect of "changing the game" is to set no boundaries. In corporate America we call this "thinking outside the box." For example, do you have interest in running a marathon? Did you automatically think of 26.2 miles and say, "No way"? I don't know your age, health, or physical condition, but let me ask, "Why not run a marathon?" If this is something you always wanted to do, start training tomorrow by walking a mile. Here's another thought: why not organize a 5K run instead to benefit a charity of your choice? Redefine marathon to what you want it to be. If I had the choice to take a red-colored magic pill that would enable me to run 26.2 miles or a blue magic pill that would enable me to organize a 5K run in my town that would also generate $2,000 for fighting world hunger, I would take the blue pill.

This is a perfect segue into the concept of giving back. As much positive energy you receive, you should strive to also give back. One way you can do this is by helping others to improve their lives. For example, I also have an interest in fighting world hunger. If I could influence the approximately 1.4 billion overweight people in the world to follow this program, they will end up also saving money because they are eating less. What if I could influence this same group of people to give back by donating just $10 a month toward fighting world hunger? That would be $168 billion dollars a year going toward world hunger. I am not sure how much money a year is needed to completely solve world hunger, but I think $168 billion a year would be a great start!

So before the critics call me nuts for steering too far off course in these last two paragraphs, here's the key message: giving back is also a great distraction strategy for working through cravings. Instead of focusing on the chocolate cake you can't eat, focus on how you can give back and help others.

Changing the game also involves applying this concept to other aspects of your life. For example, regarding small, incremental changes, do you have an unfinished project in your home because you can't find the time to accomplish it? Are you assuming that you need a free weekend to clean your garage? Imagine that instead of needing fifteen free hours on a weekend to clean your garage, you were able to put in thirty minutes six days a week? At three hours a week, your garage will be cleaned in five weeks. This approach is a lot better than having a garage be a mess for a year because you can't find a free weekend to clean it *(and for the married men, your wives will agree with me on this one!)*. Again, this is a great distraction strategy for cravings as well because it gets you moving to burn more calories while you are cleaning your garage. Make it fun, play music, dance around in the privacy of your own garage to get your heart rate elevated. Think outside the box!

The last aspect of changing the game is changing negative associations. For example, instead of me saying "bad food" in this program; I called it "real food." I do not feel guilty when eating cheeseburgers; I grew up eating cheeseburgers and still enjoy them as an adult. I also used to have a very negative association with counting calories. However, I was able to find a solution to this by educating myself on calories and just setting a calorie goal for meals and snacks. It is a lot easier for me to just focus on keeping my meals and snacks at a specific calorie value versus counting calories and wasting time entering it into a calorie tracker. Sure I had to invest a few weeks into educating myself. But remember: time flies, so these few weeks have long passed, and I now chart my meals' calorie values effortlessly.

# CHAPTER 18

# BREAKTHROUGH

As defined by the dictionary at Merriam-Webster.com, a breakthrough is "a sudden increase in knowledge, understanding, etc.: an important discovery that happens after trying for a long time to understand or explain something."[12] During my development of this program, I had several breakthroughs.

My first breakthrough was that I stopped associating diets with restrictions. Think about all of your previous failures. In addition to strong cravings, did you also feel that previous diets were too restrictive? Today's crazy-paced world demands a lot of time out of peoples' schedules. For myself, working in corporate America, I

---

12  http://www.merriam-webster.com/dictionary/breakthrough (Merriam-Webster Dictionary, Breakthrough Definition)

averaged sixty hours of work a week. Add a family with two kids in sports on top of this, and my free time for myself was minimal. As a result, a common excuse for me to quit a diet was that my job is stressful, it requires a lot of hours, and I don't have time to follow all of these food restrictions. Nor do I have the time to shop and prepare my meals. This is why I developed this program to allow your current food choices to be used as part of the program. My ability to still eat McDonald's or to get a sandwich at the deli was critical to my long-term success. And I still eat potato chips, pretzels, and cookies weekly. I was able to stop viewing these food choices as "cheating on a diet" and started viewing them as necessary calories to provide energy throughout the day.

My second breakthrough was that I changed my view on being overweight as a choice. If you really think about it, you are in control of your own choices. You can chose to not go to work tomorrow. You can choose to do something nice for someone. Guess what? You can also choose to be healthy. Being overweight or being healthy is a choice—that's it. View your current weight as an outcome of your choices on the types and quantity of foods you have consumed previously. Believe that you can choose to change your future foods and quantities to achieve happiness. The thinking that allowed me to have this breakthrough was for me to stop making excuses. I stopped blaming my work, my stress level, and my lack of will power for my failures. Then I started believing that I could make better choices in the future.

My third breakthrough was that it was more important to focus on changing my habits than it was to obtain immediate results with losing weight. I had weeks on this program where I did not lose weight or I gained weight. My archenemy (alcohol) was also at play during these weeks, which resulted in consuming lots of calories late at night. As mentioned previously, in the course of one year I did two cleanses of alcohol—going fifty days without alcohol and then later in the year going a hundred days. During these cleanse periods, I was able to change my response to stress with more exercise and meditation. I was also able to change the association that I would have more fun with my friends by drinking. In fact, I have just as much fun not drinking because it is amazing what asses people make of themselves after a few drinks. And the icing on the cake for me: one of my good friends also would not drink when we were together during my cleanses, which is a true sign of friendship.

My final breakthrough was finding out about the power of two words, "I believe." Believing truly in something does not require validation (evidence). Religion is based on these two words and some people believe in their religion so strongly, they are willing to fight to the death over their beliefs. I also believe very strongly in something: that an ordinary guy, who is not a doctor, nor trainer, nor nutritionist, can influence the industry in a new direction and make a significant impact in reducing the obesity statistics.

Here's what else I believe. I believe that everyone has the ability and power to make small incremental changes to their diet and exercise habits over time. I believe that this program will help hundreds of millions of people worldwide achieve their weight-loss goals. And most importantly I believe in you. In closing, I will leave you with a question: can you imagine what "I believe" can lead you to?

Until next time, God bless.

Harry H. Suiter was born and raised in New Jersey before going on to earn a bachelor's degree in chemistry, a master's degree in marketing, and a project management professional certification. He has over twenty years of experience in the pharmaceutical industry, having worked in various roles within research, development, and project management.

Having struggled with yo-yo dieting for over fifteen years, Suiter was inspired to write *Change Control Diet* in order to help hundreds of millions of people worldwide achieve their weight loss goals.

Suiter is married with two children.